JUS

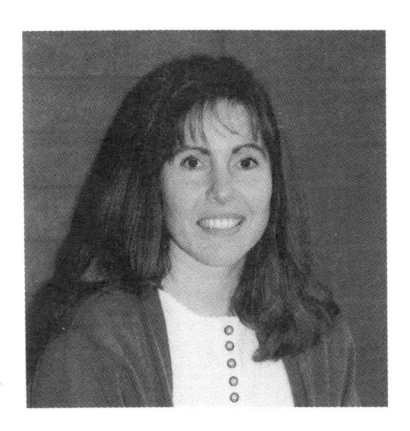

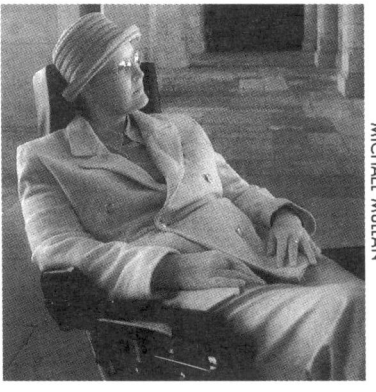

Denise Fassett MN, BHlthSc(Nsg), RN lectures at the Tasmanian School of Nursing, University of Tasmania. She was with M.R. when she suffered her first episode and followed the course of her deterioration as a nurse, a friend and a researcher.

M.R. Gallagher MSc, BSc(Hons), was a lecturer in the School of Biomedical Science, University of Tasmania, when she developed this chronic condition. She now campaigns actively in favour of voluntary euthanasia.

JUST A HEAD
Stories in a body

Denise Fassett

M.R. Gallagher

ALLEN & UNWIN

Copyright © Denise Fassett and M.R. Gallagher 1998

All rights reserved. No part of this book may be reproduced or transmitted in any form or by any means, electronic or mechanical, including photocopying, recording or by any information storage and retrieval system, without prior permission in writing from the publisher.

First published in 1998 by
Allen & Unwin
9 Atchison Street
St Leonards NSW 2065
Australia
Phone: (61 2) 8425 0100
Fax: (61 2) 9906 2218
E-mail: frontdesk@allen-unwin.com.au
Web: http://www.allen-unwin.com.au

National Library of Australia
Cataloguing-in-Publication entry:

Fassett, Denise, 1956– .
  Just a head: stories in a body.

  Bibliography.
  Includes index.
  ISBN 1 86448 565 5: $29.95.

  1. Gallagher, M. R., 1965– . 2. Patients—Australia—Biography.
  3. Medical personnel and patient—Australia—Case studies.
  4. Sick—Psychology. I. Gallagher, M. R., 1965– . II. Title.

362.1092

Set in 10.5/12 pt Goudy Old Style by DOCUPRO, Sydney
Printed by SRM Production Services, Malaysia

10 9 8 7 6 5 4 3 2 1

CONTENTS

Acknowledgments	vii
About the authors	ix
Introducing MR M.R. Gallagher	xi
1 Last day on legs	1
2 Writing the body	13
3 Reading the body	24
4 The body as text	36
5 Being 'basic nursing care'	50
6 Being unable to eat	62
7 Being 'just a head'	74
8 Lungs or legs	84
9 Being 'a psych consult'	93
10 Re-investing in science	105
11 Home at last	115
12 Being an institutionalised body	129
Reflections *Denise Fassett*	134
References	139
Index	146

ACKNOWLEDGMENTS

We would both like to thank Mary Magennis for recognising that this was a story that we could tell together. Thank you, Mary, for inspiring us with your passion for narrative and nursing, and for your guidance and support.

I would like to thank Mary Magennis, who supervised my postgraduate study when I first began to work with this story. Kim Walker sustained many 'critical conversations' with me that influenced the way in which I have engaged with the story. Thanks to Julie Cameron for support and friendship, and to Fran McInerney for reading the final draft. Thanks also to Kim Kissy and Craig McColm for helping to index the book. Special thanks to Juliet Sondermeyer, a friend and colleague, for helping me to find the space to write and for spending a few 'mad' days with me so that I could finish this project.

Matthew Fassett, Daniel Fassett and Sarah Fassett, my children, for their love and support. Stephanie Bowman and Rachel Vogelpoel, my sisters, and their families, for being there when I needed them.

Geoff Gill for love, support and friendship, and for sharing my story alongside me.

Pauline Thurlow and Gordon Thurlow, my parents, for their interest in my work and, in particular, for the very much appreciated editorial assistance.

Jocalyn Lawler for encouraging me to write this book. Judy Waters for sensitive guidance through the writing process and for having a vision of how our story could become a book.

M.R. for continuing to trust me with her words and for being the inspiration that is this story.

Denise Fassett

Thank you to Denise Fassett, my friend and co-author, for continuing interest in my story and giving me the chance to share it with others. Also, to the friends, both old and new, who have never lost faith in me and for loving me even as just a head.

I dedicate this book to the memory of my mother: my inspiration and strength.

M.R. Gallagher

ABOUT THE AUTHORS

Denise Fassett is a registered nurse and lecturer in nursing at the University of Tasmania in Launceston. She co-ordinates and teaches in the undergraduate Bachelor of Nursing programme, and also supervises Honours students. Denise completed her Master of Nursing in 1996 and hopes to enrol in a PhD in 1998. This book has grown from the thesis Denise submitted as part of her Master of Nursing studies. Her main academic interest is to continue to explore nursing and the body, and the experience of illness using narrative within a critical framework.

Denise has lived in Launceston for the past ten years with her three children. She is currently looking forward to the challenges and excitement of further study and research, and perhaps to having the chance to travel and work with others with similar interests.

M.R. Gallagher has degrees in biomedical sciences from Deakin and Melbourne Universities. She holds an MSc in Nutrition and Public Health from Deakin University and formerly taught in the School of Biomedical Science at the University of Tasmania in Launceston.

Prior to her illness, she conducted research into the relationship between bodily dimensions and diabetes, in the hope of finding an early predictor for late-onset diabetes. She received a number of small grants for this work, but was unable to pursue it due to her illness.

M.R. is enrolled in a PhD programme at RMIT University in the Department of Social Science and Social Work. Her current research is an analysis of doctor–patient relationships in those patients whose illness, such as AIDS, chronic fatigue syndrome, and other chronic or terminal illnesses, challenges the medical model. She hopes from this research to make a number of recommendations for implementation in medical education to improve these unsatisfactory relationships.

Since taking on her new life, M.R. has had to make a number of changes to her personal interests—though some remain the same. Writing is 'food for my soul' and she continues to write her story and the occasional personal article for publication. Her appetite for knowledge is voracious and when not writing, she can be found reading, or watching documentaries, or listening to the radio. Enjoying good food with good friends at a wonderful Melbourne restaurant makes a welcome break from hospital meals, and a good game of football at the MCG (especially when Carlton wins) is a great treat.

M.R.'s personal cause is for the right of people who are incurably ill and in unremitting suffering to have a good death via legalised euthanasia. She is a member and supporter of the Voluntary Euthanasia Society of Victoria.

INTRODUCING MR

M.R. Gallagher

Five years ago my life, as I knew it, was over. I was no longer an academic, a runner, a skier, or a traveller. Essentially, I became just a head. My body was gone: I was no longer a physical being. As Arthur Frank (1991) said, my body was 'colonised'. Nurses became my arms and legs. Medications control many of my physiological and biochemical systems. Doctors make decisions about my body.

In your young adult years you feel invincible. You never think of illness, death or dying. Certainly everything seemed to be coming together for me and my life was taking on a definite shape. I was a young academic at the University of Tasmania and on the verge of a good promotion. My research was beginning to attract funding. I was renovating my own house. I had travelled extensively. My training was getting back on track after a badly fractured ankle. The ski season had been great. Also, I had so many hopes, dreams and aspirations. I intended to return to study and complete a medical degree. Africa was next on my travel list. The Hawaii Ironman competition was my long-term training goal. I dreamed of skiing every continent. My health was good and, apart from mild asthma, I had never really been sick. It seemed that life could not have been better.

This all changed with one single asthma attack whilst out training with my friend Denise on a frosty Tasmanian morning in late September 1992. It was a warning that I never heeded. I think

I saw it as a mere interruption, an inconvenience. In fact I had many warnings that I chose to ignore, as I had required more and more Ventolin during training for some time. I was still attached to intravenous lines and needing copious quantities of drugs, when I started thinking about getting back to work and wondering when I could get back into my training. I got better, out of hospital and as soon as I could I was back at work, into the training and even went to Perth for a conference. Just six weeks later I was to walk for the very last time. I had another asthma attack whilst out training and found myself unable to breathe and in intensive care.

This was the start of my new life and as my body lost more functions and thus became even more taken over by medicine or even more 'colonised', I found myself becoming just a head. I was no longer a person but 'the asthmatic' in Bed 1. Doctors took over control of my body and any decisions made about it. Initially, I had respiratory failure from severe asthma but as time passed it seemed that something else had gone seriously wrong with my body. This started a flurry of tests and investigations. There was great interest in me for a time, it was a challenge to find Bed 1 a diagnosis. However, eventually Bed 1 was forgotten by medicine as it continued to frustrate efforts to fit its problem into a neat medical pigeon-hole. There were many pieces to the puzzle but no permutation or combination could form a recognisable picture. Thus, the body, devastated by this mystery illness, was also shunned.

I found myself in the medical wilderness of the psychosomatic. The doctors didn't know what was wrong with me, therefore it must have been all in my head. The person in me was now recognised but nothing was done to help as apparently it was my own fault. I was now somehow outside the doctors' control, I couldn't be treated in a traditional way or told I had a terminal illness and therefore my relationship with the medical staff ended. Once it had been written in my progress notes that I was 'for a psych consult' I felt further marginalised and, at times, even vilified. I felt much frustration and anger that the doctor never, in six weeks, examined me. He didn't look at my incredibly wasted body or even listen to the chest of the asthmatic. He could only stand at the end of my bed and stare at me or ask me inane questions such as *'Are you walking yet?'* or *'What do you think is wrong with you?'*. Although my breathing had improved somewhat I was losing more and more control over my body. The functions that I lost were taken over by the nurses on my ward as if in silent conspiracy with my illness.

Introducing MR

I have never felt more alone and frightened in my life. My medical knowledge didn't help me and in some ways it taunted me. It seemed no-one could help me. I knew that something catastrophic had happened to my body but no-one was doing anything to help me. I didn't ever even see a psychiatrist. Escape to Melbourne was my only chance.

With the help of friends I organised to be airlifted to a large teaching hospital in Melbourne. I think the doctors in Launceston were pleased that I was going as I would no longer be their problem. In preparing the usual doctor transfer letter my doctor finally looked at me and examined me for himself. There was no excuse not to. They saw how exhausted I was; how wasted my runner's legs were; blood gas results told them that there was a problem with my breathing. There were questions and my story was beginning to have some credibility again. However it was too little, too late: I was out of there.

Once I was in hospital in Melbourne I was assaulted with a barrage of tests and investigations. Every specialty from infectious diseases to haematology visited my bedside with a plethora of questions. I was stuck in machines and machines were stuck in me. I felt almost desperate for a diagnosis. The neurologist's first impression was that I had Guillain-Barré Syndrome but subsequent testing failed to confirm this. As I was presenting such a conundrum to the doctors I was presented to a grand round and even though I was clothed I felt naked to the inquiring stares of the crowded audience. Ultimately, it couldn't be decided exactly what it was that was wrong with me. There was no mention of it being a psychosomatic condition but it was difficult not knowing what condition I had. It was decided that I should now go into rehabilitation and with therapy I would get better. That was the main thing really, to get better. I always thought I would and couldn't wait to get back to my old life. I had just over three months until University started again and I was determined to be there.

I faced the rehabilitation hospital with both hope and trepidation. Hope for recovery; trepidation regarding how distant I now felt from my body. It felt so weak, so strange, so awkward, yet I had to make it mine again in order to get my beloved life back. I had so much incentive to reclaim my body but it wasn't to be enough. Everything I had I put into my therapy but before long I started to realise that it just wasn't working. I couldn't find the energy, the control that I needed. After three months the rehabilitation staff decided that I had to leave because I wasn't getting any better. Again I found myself bewildered and lonely. How could I go home like this? I couldn't look after myself yet I wasn't given a choice.

Back home to Tasmania I went. Being back at home was a disaster. I couldn't get the support services that I needed and my house was unsuitable for a disabled person. Before long I found myself back in hospital in a much weakened condition. My breathing had deteriorated, I had lost all my hard fought for gains and I was malnourished and dehydrated. The testing and investigations started again to no avail. At least I was treated like a sick body this time. Still, I don't think that the doctors knew what to do with me so I was put in the rehabilitation ward. By this stage a diagnosis was no longer important to me, what was important was to get better. My faith in medicine was shattered, but my determination to get well had hardly wavered and I threw myself into whatever I had to do to achieve this. Tube feeding re-nourished me, antibiotics treated my infections, new medications stabilised my condition and I put my all into physiotherapy, occupational therapy and speech therapy. I became healthier and stable but physically not much better. It seemed impossible to reclaim my body. The conspiracy continued: my illness had seemingly given my arms and legs permanently to the nurses who cared for me.

In early September 1993 the bombshell was dropped. During a meeting with my therapists and doctors I was told by a doctor that I would never get better. More than that, I was told that I would never be able to work or be able to do anything else that was useful, and I would have to live in a nursing home. I was stunned. It just couldn't be true. So I found myself going into survival mode. I fought so hard to stay out of a nursing home and succeeded in moving back home with attendant carers to look after me. They would become my new arms and legs. I decided if the medical system wouldn't help me to get better then I would just have to do it myself.

Going home proved much harder than I would ever admit to the system which told me I was doomed to fail if I lived at home. I was given only four hours a day of care to meet all my needs. It wasn't enough time but I had no choice but to survive with these hours. My carers were great but they couldn't stop me from getting sick. I had fifteen hospital admissions in twelve months. I was always getting infections: in my bladder, kidneys, lungs, or stoma.

Introducing MR

My asthma was out of control and I ended up on enteral feeding. Things got worse and worse as time went on and I no longer had any well days; I was in constant pain. On a personal level I suffered many blows: I had to sell my beloved house; I lost my job and research money and I couldn't even study. It seemed that life could just not have been any worse. I was headed for renal and respiratory failure but there was no way I was going to be kept alive by machines in a nursing home.

There was no choice: I had to die. My life had no quality and I faced only continued and worsening illness. Soon I would be unable to do anything. My eyesight was so bad I couldn't even watch the mindless television. I told my doctor: he called a psychiatrist. The psychiatrist couldn't disagree with me or find any evidence of endogenous depression. I called my friends: they gathered around to say goodbye. I received many letters and calls of love and support. Beautiful flowers adorned my room. My final act was to take a flight in a light aircraft over the magnificent mountains of Northern Tasmania with some friends.

Late January 1995 I stopped my medication and enteral feeding, and even the small amount of fluid I drank. A friend removed my hated feeding tube. A few friends stayed with me as I set out on my journey to the next life. Two days later my doctor broke into my house via the kitchen window and offered me the world. He promised to send me to the spinal unit in Melbourne to have my medical problems sorted out and then on to specialised rehabilitation to connect with all the latest technology to give me back some quality of life. He had a promise for everything. It was too tempting. I didn't want to die if there were some chance of being well again and be able to do things, even if it was only reading. Intravenous fluids were started but a day later I was unconscious and in hospital. I certainly hadn't done my already weakened body any good by dehydrating it for three days. I didn't leave hospital for nearly two years.

My doctor didn't, or couldn't, keep his promise. He made a promise he hadn't looked into and it was just not a possibility. I felt so betrayed by him and angry with myself for believing him, a doctor. Something had to be done, so again I relied on my friends for help in getting back to Melbourne to see the specialists I needed. I was airlifted to Melbourne on 14 February 1995 and again entered the merry-go-round of the medical system. I had all the tests and investigations and was visited by all the specialists. I was supposed to be there for seven days but stayed for six weeks: I was apparently so interesting. However, this time after two and a half years I had a diagnosis: Post Intensive Care Neuropathy. I had never heard of it and neither had anyone else except the Professor. It didn't change anything much as there was no treatment or cure. Rehabilitation, again, was the answer: long-term rehabilitation. The trouble was no-one wanted to take the wasted, catheterised Biafran that I had become. I would take too much care and my rehabilitation would be too long. I felt extremely unwanted.

Eventually a place was found: a small, obscure private hospital in the inner suburbs which took long-term rehabilitation patients. I think the only reason they agreed to take me was for the money. The ward I was on was drab and unkempt and the air was punctuated with crazed and demented wails and shouts and smelled badly of urine and faeces. I was instantly reminded of *One Flew Over the Cuckoo's Nest*. Where was it that I had been dumped? But there was no choice. The saving grace of the ward was the fantastic nursing staff who did their best to make me at home. I was still met with curious gazes as I looked so malnourished and unwell and sported a bald head from drug therapy. It seemed that I was still to be an enigma. I certainly didn't have an easy time at this place especially with the CEO taking an instant dislike to me and taking every opportunity to make my life difficult. The therapists were also unsure of me and didn't know what to do with my floppy, wasted, elongated body. So they didn't do anything and left me to the various students who came to work on the ward who admittedly did their best for me. I made some gains with improvements in my neck strength and some arm movements, however fatigue and pain limited me severely. It was never enough though and after twelve months, and $160 000, my private health insurance would no longer pay for me to stay in hospital. Feelings of isolation and desperation overtook me. What was to happen to me now? It seemed I was destined for that nursing home I promised myself I would never go to.

In September 1996 I entered a nursing home in inner Melbourne. I couldn't believe that I was going and I felt so sad for so many things. This symbolised the pinnacle of my losses and signalled a point of no return. I was filled with trepidation at being confronted with new sets of arms and legs. I have always hated training people to look after me—it is such an effort. My friend Shirley brought me to the home and I cried all the way there in

Introducing MR

the taxi. I couldn't go inside so she had to wheel me. Meanwhile, I had managed to compose myself to face this new devil. The staff seemed friendly enough, but I wasn't really interested. The only saving grace of the place was I had my own spacious room in which to closet myself. The goodbye, when Shirley left me after setting up my room, was one of the hardest in my life. My melancholy was overwhelming.

With time I did settle in; I got used to the staff and now spend the majority of time in my room with my voice-activated computer (which Macintosh had helped me to purchase). My computer has become the centre of my life as it brings me the world and provides my mind with the freedom and stimulation that it needs. My body however has continued to deteriorate and I am still plagued by infections, fatigue, and severe pain. The doctor I had didn't appreciate my pain and eventually I saw less and less of him as he lost interest, so I got a doctor who was more in tune with my situation. After three months in the nursing home, the euthanasia debate was starting to heat up and I felt compelled to share my story to hopefully give the public some insight to the life that people can face. More importantly, my life had reached a point where I started to explore my options for dying. The pain was unbearable and I guess I was frightened of my unknown future and what it might hold. I didn't and don't want to die fighting for every breath or attached to some machine. I explored my options with known euthanasia doctors and Philip Nitschke took an interest in my case. I had hoped, when I was ready, to access the *Rights of the Terminally Ill Act* in the Northern Territory but parliament took that option away from me. The only way I could die prematurely is with the help of someone else, which I am not prepared to do for the trouble it could cause for my helper. I have made provisions with the *Refusal of Medical Treatment Act* of 1988 which prevents anyone from taking heroic measures to keep me alive. If I find myself rapidly deteriorating then I will return to my original plan of dehydrating myself to death.

As for the present, I still maintain my just a head existence. I have sought solutions to my pain but there is little that can be done without compromising my breathing or diminishing the sharpness of my still active mind. My head is so important to me, and helps to distract me from the pain by meditation or work on my computer. A recent visit to a neurologist has shed more light on my condition which is an inflammatory neuropathy—which basically means that it is progressive. I always thought that I would get worse with time but not due to a disease process. So my medical future is not that bright as my breathing and eyesight have started to be affected and my pain only promises to get worse. On a personal front I am lucky to have many wonderful friends who give me the love and support that I need. I am also lucky that I enjoy my own company and spend many of my waking hours working on my computer.

Boredom is not a problem as I have been kept busy with writing which gives me so much joy now. Many of my friends live overseas, so I write many letters, usually via e-mail and I also keep up with current research via the Internet. Hopefully, my plans to do a PhD, where I can explore the doctor–patient relationship, will be realised. This book has also kept me busy and has certainly been a cathartic experience as I have relived and faced much of what has happened to me during my new life. It has also helped me to grieve my beloved old life. The book has also been the impetus to other writings and I continue to tell my story which will only end when I am faced with my next life.

1

LAST DAY ON LEGS

> *Illness is the night side of life, a more onerous citizenship. Everyone who is born holds dual citizenship, in the kingdom of the well and in the kingdom of the sick. Although we all prefer to use only the good passport, sooner or later each of us is obliged, at least for a spell, to identify ourselves as citizens of that other place.* (Susan Sontag 1990, p. 3)

BECOMING FRIENDS

As a person I have, from time to time, identified myself as a 'citizen of the kingdom of the sick' (Sontag 1990, p. 3). However, like many people my experiences of being ill have been transitory and I spend most of my time as a well person. I have spent all of my working life as a nurse, and it has been in this role that I have come to know illness through the experiences of others who live out their lives 'in that other place' as described by Sontag (1990, p. 3). This book is about living in the kingdom of the sick. Through the story of a young woman, whose name is MR, I explore some of her experiences of being ill. I was with MR when she crossed that boundary that seems to exist between illness and wellness, when her story of living in the kingdom of the sick began. It seems appropriate then to begin this book with the story of our first meeting and of how MR became ill.

Every few years I look in the mirror and think 'this is the year of the diet'. The year I met MR was one of those years. That year I was determined to be very thin. I think I had developed what Wolf (1990, p. 186) refers to as a 'fear of fat'. In a determined effort to change my body I succumbed to the stereotypical images of other women's bodies in order to be described as feminine and thin. It was not hard to find another woman whose body was, as Bordo (1989, p. 28) suggested, 'a site of struggle' like mine—someone caught in the same web of a cultural conspiracy which constrains and regulates women's bodies; someone who would exercise and diet with me to change her body.

After MR and I met we recognised in each other a similar struggle, a struggle that many women share, born of a desire to look a particular way.

This struggle with our bodies was an important issue for both of us because it formed the basis of our friendship. Without that we were perhaps two unlikely friends because MR is a scientist and I am a nurse and we did not have many shared understandings about the world. This was later to change but, at the time, it was our absolute commitment to diet and exercise that brought us together. The irony of all of this was that neither of us ever imagined that MR's body and her whole life were about to change dramatically and that her experiences would impact on and shape both of our lives so intensely.

MR: I had just come out of plaster because of a fractured ankle when I decided to get fit again. I was extremely unfit and had put on some abhorrent body weight. I enjoyed talking to Denise on those early morning strolls when we had lively debates on many philosophical issues. Denise and I are both what I would describe as headstrong characters but we are very different from each other. Despite our differences I think we respected each other's opinions. I learnt a great deal on those cold frosty mornings as our conversations introduced me to a whole new world of thinking.

Asthma was to prove our nemesis. Until then my asthma had been no more than a minor irritation. I refused to acknowledge the insidious nature of asthma and I was non-compliant with my medications. I never accepted that asthma was a serious problem but just an aberration which I thought that I had control over.

LAST DAY ON LEGS

We knew very little about each other when we first decided to walk early each morning. I did know MR had asthma and that she seemed well informed on her condition and her treatment. We walked every day on cold frosty mornings in the dark. We lived in Launceston, a picturesque country town nestled in amongst the hills. We sometimes welcomed those hills (and there were many) to warm us up and to burn up that excess fat. Yes, I admit, we were obsessional but we were caught in the 'tyranny of slenderness' and all of the 'normalising' self-disciplinary practices that go with that (Bordo 1990).

I think we became friends during this time because we had 'critical' conversations about our desire to change our bodies and the way each of us constructed being a woman. I was reading *The Beauty Myth*, savouring Naomi Wolf's every word of 'fear of fat'. We would intellectualise, theorise and analyse what we were doing but still relentlessly pursued that very myth. Nothing deterred us from our early morning walks—even MR's asthma. As she would say, she lived with asthma rather than being an asthmatic.

As we plunged into the depths of a very cold Launceston winter MR began to use her inhaler more often and we discussed the possibility of her having an asthma attack while we were walking. It isn't only the cold that you have to consider in Launceston. There is also the thick smoke that gets trapped in the valley overnight from the many slow-burning wood heaters used there. MR insisted that she was well prepared and she wore a small pouch to store her medications. However, one morning MR was hospitalised with acute asthma after one of our walks. I thought the walks would stop after that but MR talked of getting out of hospital and getting going again. It certainly gave us both a scare but MR was not about to give up exercise. Her medications were reviewed and altered and we decided to walk after work when the air was much warmer. The time it took for MR to recover gave the weather a chance to warm up and we were able to enjoy many more walks as we chatted endlessly and unravelled our life stories to each other.

One particularly warm afternoon we ventured out intending to take our time on a much longer walk. This time we had a friend, Julie, with us and I remember how we laughed so much that when we started out on our walk people glanced at us as they passed us by. We decided to walk through the Cataract Gorge because it is quite spectacular and close to where we live. In the winter we had walked over the suspension bridge and watched the white water thunder under us engulfing the green lawns and the swimming pool. Peacock calls fill the air and there is a strange mixture of European trees that give way to native bush. Near to the suspension bridge is a walk that winds high above the river through the bush to an old power station called Duck Reach.

I had mixed feelings about walking to Duck Reach on this particular day because it was near there that MR had her first asthma attack. I remember glancing at MR before we made our way along the track. I think we even raised the issue of the possibility of her having an asthma attack somewhere remote. Lulled into a false sense of security by the warmth of the afternoon we decided to continue. We were going to walk back along the road once we got to the power station which was about two kilometres away. We walked slowly because it really is very beautiful along the track and every now and then stopped to take in the view.

After about twenty minutes of walking and not far from the power station, MR suddenly seemed troubled, not short of breath, just uneasy. We stopped and MR said that she was experiencing difficulty in breathing and swallowing. I was scared because of the last experience with her and now here we were on a fairly remote track with quite a climb to the nearest phone. We sat on a bridge for a few minutes and then MR said that she was feeling much better and insisted that she could walk home.

MR: I don't really remember any of this. I do remember having increasing difficulty in breathing and holding onto reality. I desperately wanted to ignore what was happening to me and ultimately my pig-headedness made it worse.

I was pleased that Julie was with us to help make the decision to continue walking. As soon as we were well away from any houses MR became troubled again. We slowly walked MR towards the nearest house and help. There was silence—no one spoke as we walked up the road because we all knew we had made an unfortunate decision to go on. When we got to the first sign of houses Julie went for help. MR was sitting down now and she seemed to get worse. I was scared, and I could hear my voice telling MR to relax while another voice inside me was yelling for Julie to come back quickly with help. Julie came back and help soon arrived. The hospital, only a few minutes away, is very visible from most vantage points in Launceston and was a welcome sight as it came into view from the hill where we were being driven down.

This was the last day that MR ever walked again and so her life, as she knew it, changed in that instant. On the way to the hospital Julie and I finally looked at each other as we became relaxed enough to acknowledge our fear. We arrived at the hospital and within minutes MR was lying on a trolley in accident and emergency having an intravenous line inserted. MR seemed to get worse in the hospital and the staff quickly responded. Nurses were drawing up drugs, machines were plugged in and scanned for information and doctors were examining her. It all seemed so unreal to me—one minute we had been walking and laughing and now MR was fighting for her every breath.

There was a sudden decision that MR should be transferred to the intensive care unit (ICU) and one of the nurses handed me her shoes. I followed the trolley along the corridor and only had time to thrust the shoes under the trolley, and to give MR what I hoped was an encouraging look before she disappeared through some double doors. I cannot remember leaving the hospital or where Julie was, or even how I got home. I was shocked because I had not expected MR to go to ICU. I was trying to make sense of what had happened, going over every moment and thinking did I do the right thing? I reassured myself that MR would be stabilised very quickly and discharged in next to no time. She is a strong woman, I thought, she will bounce back—but she never did.

WHY THIS STORY?

At the time that MR and I first met I was a lecturer and a postgraduate student in nursing, deeply immersed in a critique of the philosophy of science. Everything that I read moved me further and further away from the shackles of positivism that had constrained the health science degree I had undertaken previously. When I timidly dangled my toes into the critical social sciences, poststructuralism and postmodernism, it is true to say that I started to think about knowledge and meaning being constituted through language and the body and I was drawn to more unconventional ways of exploring nursing. Since then, when I read or write about nursing, MR always comes to mind. Her incredible chronicle of experience makes me aware that her life and her experiences are not only reflected in these stories but also have actually been created through them.

Through MR's experiences of being ill I found that I was confronted with 'the body' and how it is theoretically approached in nursing. My interest in the body led me to Jocalyn Lawler's book *Behind the Screens: Nursing, Somology, and the Problem of the Body* (1991). Her work has had a profound impact on the way I now think about nursing and on how I interrogated nursing as a postgraduate student. I can best describe this experience as 'freeing'. It provided me with the intellectual stimulus to explore aspects of nursing that I had previously avoided or chosen to ignore.

Lawler (1991, p. vi) proposes that 'the body [is] the pivotal construct which [has] the capacity to explain lots of things about nursing as an occupation'. In explicating a theory of the body she suggests that 'nursing practice is fundamentally about people's experiences of embodied existence, particularly at those times when the body fails to function normally' (Lawler 1991, p. vi). I was beginning to understand what nursing meant to me through the connections I had made between MR's experiences of her body and my experiences of nursing. I wanted to know more about her experiences of her embodied existence as an ill woman over the last few years. Because I was a student at this time it seemed a natural progression to formalise my interest in MR's story in the form of a study. This was how MR and I first came to work together with her story.

I spoke with MR about my interest in exploring her story for my Masters thesis. Even though as a researcher and scientist she would have been interested to examine possible 'causes' to explain her illness, she was interested in my suggested approach. I discussed how I wanted to use narrative (or story telling) as a method to engage us both in critical conversations around her illness experiences. I knew that MR was familiar with and respected the work of Oliver Sacks and we had conversations around some of his ideas that helped to motivate us both to explore the notion of narrative and the experiences of illness. MR clearly wanted to tell her story as no one had ever really asked her to do that before, not even me.

MR: When Denise first approached me about me telling my story I was chuffed that someone was actually interested. I thought that critically analysing my story would shed some light onto my illness experiences. It was also an opportunity to share my story with someone who had the capacity for empathy and understanding. These two factors have been conspicuous by their absence throughout my illness. I remembered reading in one of Sacks' books that one should ask not what disease the person has, but what person has the disease.

MR knew that I had become interested in her experiences of embodiment and that she thought of herself as a mind and a body. I had actually heard her describe herself as 'just a head'. I wondered how nurses went about caring for someone who saw themselves as just a head and what it might be like to abandon your own body. It was the next few sentences that MR spoke that profoundly influenced and shaped my study and later this book.

Denise: So how would you describe yourself now?

MR: I guess I am really 'just a head'.

Denise: How do nurses go about caring for someone who sees themselves 'just as a head'?

MR: I guess I care for my head and everyone cares for everything else.

Denise: So are you saying that you care for your mind and others care for your body?

MR: Yes, I'm not saying that nurses picked me out to treat me either *not as* a person or *as* a person, but some nurses seem to treat all of their patients as people and a lot of nurses treat *none* of their patients as people. Before I was ill I was very aware of my body, but being ill has forced me to split my body and mind. I've given up my body to be cared for because I have no control over it but I feel I have absolute control over my mind.

THE CARTESIAN BODY

Clearly, MR is talking about her body as an object—a body aware of itself because it does not function and aware of itself because of having things done to it. According to Leder (1984, p. 33) the process of objectifying the body is often begun by the illness itself. Referring to Strauss (1963), Leder (1984, p. 33) argues that 'when suffering the body can come to appear as Other'. It is the Cartesian body, the mechanical body, the body which houses biological processes that becomes ill. Once a person presents his or her body for physical examination the immediate task is to search for the disease—this forces a person like MR to experience her body as a scientific object. In wellness bodies are usually taken for granted and as a result embodiment is also taken for granted.

Cartesian, as I will explain later, is a term associated with René Descartes who is considered by many to be the founder of modern philosophy. According to Capra (1982, p. 42) the basis of Cartesian philosophy is a belief in the certainty of scientific knowledge. As a mathematician, Descartes' contribution to science, through analytical reasoning as a method, has proved to be extremely successful. However, this method when introduced into the life sciences led him to conclude that mind and matter are both separate and different. Capra (1982, p. 45) argues that this philosophy has created endless confusion about the relationship between mind and matter and has actually prevented 'doctors from seriously considering the psychological dimensions of illness, and psychotherapists from dealing with their [sic] patients' bodies'.

Nurses may come across reference to Descartes if they are reading contemporary nursing scholarship. Unfortunately it has been my experience with nursing students that they are usually very confused as to the significance of the profound influence of Descartes' work on Western thought and thus nursing. These students, as with most people, have been encouraged throughout their lives to consider living organisms as machines—a critique of this highlights the severe limitations of science in general and this makes them feel uncomfortable. They also get frustrated because transcending the Cartesian view of the body is almost impossible with the language that most people use and understand.

My experiences of learning about Descartes as a nurse came about when I was a postgraduate student and my lecturer introduced me to Bernstein (1983). This book along with Capra (1982), Kuhn (1970), Chalmers (1976) and Charlesworth (1982) set me on a pathway that confronted many of my beliefs. At first I thought it was enough to question what I believed and to recognise some of the problems in health that I might encounter as a nurse. It was not until MR became ill that for the first time I was really able to see how someone's life is actually shaped by these beliefs. It was only when I began to examine MR's story that I began to understand how Capra (1982) could believe that clinging to a mechanistic world view has brought us perilously close to destruction.

MR made sense of her body as a scientific object to be understood as was clearly evident in the way MR spoke of the duality of her mind and body. The language through which MR made sense of her body constitutes the nature of her illness and the illness experience itself. MR talked about having to become dualistic about herself as a response to being ill. In her words *'being ill has forced me to split my mind from my body'*.

The medical profession also successfully separated MR into a mind and a body. When they had exhausted all of the possible scientific explanations searching for a diagnosis they said that her condition was psychosomatic in origin. Psychosomatic is a term used in medicine to imply there is a mind and a body and that a problem in or with the mind can 'cause' a problem in the body. There is nothing unusual about this, considering we know that the epistemological tradition of Cartesian dualism has dominated the way the body has been understood in medicine and nursing (Scheper-Hughes and Lock 1987). But what do we know about what this might mean to a person living through an illness? How legitimate does a person feel if their illness is attributed to a psychosomatic state? Listening to MR describe herself, in terms that forced her mind and body apart, was confronting for me as a nurse because it forced me to think about how significant language was in shaping people's experiences of their bodies. Moreover, it was the ease with which MR separated mind from matter that so unsettled me.

Illness is a time when people experience the profound consequences of being a medicalised Cartesian body. Indeed, it is extremely difficult to move beyond notions of the 'medicalised' body because of the way illness is constructed through Cartesian understandings. Frank (1990, p. 132) argues that science and the way it influences our understandings of the body, both contradict and complicate theorising the body and that 'our capacity to experience the body directly, or theorise it indirectly, is inextricably medicalised' (Frank 1990, p. 136).

Parker (1991a, p. 304) points out, however, that the consequences of the widespread acceptance of these science-based assumptions have 'resulted in an understanding of the body as an object of medical scrutiny and of technical intervention and of health as the absence of disease'. Nursing scholars are now beginning to critique such dominant scientific assumptions of the body and to recognise how scientific attitudes are problematic for nursing and health care because they are not congruent with notions of the human world of nursing and health care (Parker 1991a; Taylor 1994).

I believe that the difficulty nurses have in terms of re-thinking the body is that they continue to reinforce a dualistic and mechanistic approach in their practices. Handovers, nursing notes, nursing rituals and routines, ward rounds, and more recently the Australian Nursing Council Incorporated (ANCI) competencies are all a testimony to the objectification of the body in nursing (see Parker and Gardner 1991–92, 1992; Parker, Gardner and Wiltshire 1992; Street 1992a and b; Walker 1993, 1994a, 1994b, 1995). This creates a paradox if you believe, as I do, that the body is central to nursing as a discipline. It is surely then an imperative for nursing to re-think the 'body' or as Lawler (1991, p. 227) suggests to 'build a theory of the body' if nursing is ever to be part of the challenge to move beyond mechanistic reductionist views of health.

In response to what MR was experiencing I wanted to find a way to re-think the body, to deepen my understandings of the lived experiences of illness and suffering and to translate these understandings in the way in which I teach the problem of the body to nurses. The experience of illness is the 'stuff' of nursing. Nurses listen to and share the intimate life stories of the people with whom they interact every day. As Walker (1993, p. 173) reminds us, nurses 'must listen to and share the stories of outrage and disbelief, the tales of abjection and torture, the narratives of disquietude and despair, and the histories of struggles with pain and impending death'. It is through these stories that I believe that nurses discover what for me has always been 'intuitively clear and now is becoming formally clear, that we are in no sense machines or impersonal automata' (Sacks 1984, p. 188).

Through my experiences as a postgraduate student and this friendship, I began to search through narrative techniques for a legitimate space to bring to the surface what I believe has always been known but hidden in the oral culture of nursing. I was challenged with finding a way to give MR voice to her experiences. Following Judy Lumby (1992) I wanted to explore story telling as a methodology for nurses. Lumby (1992) spent almost two and a half years sharing stories with one woman who had a life-threatening illness and who, like MR and I, were friends and co-researchers.

I had heard Lumby speak to her research and was inspired because her work was accessible to me as a nurse, as a woman, and as an academic. Story telling is a familiar way through which women communicate with each other every day and many nurses are familiar with story telling because of the oral culture that exists in nursing. As an academic Lumby argues that storytelling is an exciting possibility as a mode of research moving away from the boundaries of conventional research and this idea both scared and motivated me at the same time (Lumby 1992).

THE STORY OF ONE

Lumby's work was indeed, as she suggests a 'new space' in which to explore women's experiences and thoughts (Lumby 1992, p. 12). When I began my research people would ask 'how many participants were in the study?' Lumby gave me the courage, then the pleasure, to be able to say, 'one'. I thought that story telling, as a research approach, had some exciting possibilities for the production of knowledge because it cuts across the traditional nature of objective research. Story telling could be 'interactive, contextualised and humanely compelling through the recognition that 'knowledge is socially constituted, historically embedded, and valuationally based' (Lather 1991, p. 52).

So as I begin to reveal MR's story through the pages of this book I feel I should make explicit some of the complexity of such an endeavour because there is not just one story to tell. There are many stories and, as they run alongside each other, twist and turn, intersect and join, they are sometimes me, sometimes MR, and sometimes 'other' to both of us. Frank (1991, p. 50) writes 'How medicine treats the body is an essential part of the story of illness, but it is never more than half of the story. The other half is the body itself'. I have attempted to bring together these stories to make the body central through MR's experiences.

When I talk of MR's experiences I am not implying that her experiences can be generalised but rather that her unique experiences may speak to others through a certain and necessary celebration of 'difference'. MR's story has challenged me to 'write the body'. I hope that those who read this will be provoked into telling their own stories of embodiment and that, in time, there will be stories which offer a range of different positions on the problematic of illness and the body. I further hope that it will become clearer how narrative may shape and construct our lives and thus our reality.

2

WRITING THE BODY

MANY BODIES

In the next two chapters I spend time problematising the body and making connections with and between narrative and notions of 'body', thus revealing something new about our understandings of the body generally. Benoist and Cathebras (1993, p. 857) argue that the concepts and notions of the body in the literature are so diverse that an analysis of the literature is almost impossible. This was reassuring to read because, as I travel through the theorists writing the body, there are many 'bodies' to consider from the prescientific body, to the postmodern body. Thus as more theorists attempt to re-situate the body they have created an endless maze of typologies. McLaren (1988, p. 57) argues that the term 'body' is problematic by his following remarks. 'The term "body" is a promiscuous term that ranges wildly from being understood as a warehouse of archaic instinctual drives, to a cauldron of seething libidinal impulses, to a phallocentric economy waging war on women, to a lump of perishable matter, to a fiction of discourse'.

THE BODY

Much of the theoretical work around the body follows McLaren's (1988) view that the body can be constructed as 'a fiction of discourse' (see Bordo 1989, 1990, 1993; Foucault 1965, 1973, 1976, 1977, 1980; Silverman 1984; Frank 1991; McLaren 1988; Scheper-Hughes and Lock 1987; Wilcox *et al.* 1990; and Butler 1993) or as a 'phallocentric economy waging war on women' (see Grosz 1992, 1994; Cixous 1981). Bryan Turner (1992, p. 16), a sociologist, who has produced some of the major studies on the body talks about 'having a body', 'being a body', and 'doing a body'. Using a comparative and historical approach, the body is conceived by Turner (1984) as a potentiality which is elaborated by culture and developed in social relations.

Turner (1992, p. 18) has been interested in the concept of the body as a target of many diverse social practices which aim at regulating the body and, in particular, the regulation of female sexuality. Frank (1990, p. 134) argues that to date Turner provides the most coherent sociological theory of the body but adds that Turner has become 'less sure of what a body is' as his work has progressed. Foucault (1973, 1965, 1977) analysed medicine, psychiatry and criminal justice to examine how 'bodies' are produced by discourses which were to produce power/knowledge over bodies. This analysis has been particularly relevant to nursing because it highlights the tension that exists when one 'acknowledges that we are both victims and agents within systems of domination' (Sawicki 1991, p. 10).

As contemporary scholars are engaging with the term 'body' there are many debates emerging as to which discipline best accommodates the body; Frank (1990, p. 131) comments, 'bodies are in, in academia as well as in popular culture'. There is an academic scramble to theorise the body and to thus lay claim to particular truths that will, in time, construct different experiences for people and their bodies. It is an exciting time in that respect. But also it is a time when I cannot help but be concerned that, in the rush to theoretically accommodate bodies, the relationship between 'real bodies' and the body as constructed in discourses may be lost (McLaren 1988). Moreover, even though there is an endless array of categories that classify the body, I do not believe that we, as yet, have adequately theorised what it means to be 'a lump of perishable matter' (McLaren 1988, p. 57) or that which I call the Cartesian body. This must come before we can begin to understand the concept of 'real bodies' explicated by Silverman (1983) in (McLaren 1988, p. 59).

EMBODIMENT IN NURSING THROUGH THE RHETORIC OF ILLNESS

In nursing scholarship Lawler (1991, p. 3) argues that the body's presence has been 'implicit, subsumed and privatised'. This is interesting because in nursing practice the body is very explicit. All disciplines, it would seem, are faced with the 'problem of the body'. But Lawler (1991, p. 3) argues that 'nursing can, and does necessarily and inevitably accommodate the body and corporeal existence' in ways that most other disciplines do not. Lawler (1991) further argues that nursing is in a prime position to theorise the body because of the knowledges nurses can generate through their sustained intimate contact with people and their bodies.

However, nurses are predominantly women and in theorising the body, they are challenged with writing a theory that does not obscure gender and 'provides women with non-patriarchal terms for representing themselves' (Grosz 1994, p. 188). Grosz (1994, p. 3) remarks that 'feminism has uncritically adopted many philosophical assumptions regarding the role of the body which are complicit in the misogyny which characterises Western thought'.

Nurses' constructions of the body have been reviewed more recently by Colin Holmes (1994). Holmes (1994, p. 116) argues that current scholarship on the body in nursing signals 'recognition that the body, and the discourses which it invokes, have been recognised as a central concern to nursing'. He continues by saying that he considers the 'field relatively untouched' (Holmes 1994, p. 116). Holmes discusses Lawler's work and makes the comment that 'the most valuable aspect of Lawler's text of 1992 has been to expose the regimes of the body as they affect both the clinical practices and the discourses of nursing' (Holmes 1994, p. 116). Many nurse clinicians speak of the alienation and distance they feel when they are exposed to nursing scholarship. By making the body explicit Lawler's (1991) work does seem to engage these nurses with a certain interest as they recognise the centrality of the body to their nursing practice.

This was highlighted for me during a conversation with some clinical nurses. Many of these registered nurses had read Lawler's (1991) work as part of their university studies. Knowing that these students, who were registered nurses, were thinking about the body, for the first time in my teaching I was able to discuss with them my interest in the body through MR's and my experiences. I remember their interest, the connections they all made between Lawler's work and their current nursing practice, and their enthusiasm to narrate their stories about embodiment in illness. As I talked about how MR experienced being ill there was a silence—but it was a knowing silence. The nurses were as uncomfortable as I was with the way MR described herself through her story as just a head.

Later as I reflected I realised that MR's story exposed and confronted nurses with the full impact of how Cartesian reductive thinking shapes peoples' illness experiences. The nurses had difficulty with MR's story because their rhetoric of holism collided with the mechanistic constructions of the body that dominated MR's experience of illness. In fact from this discussion we critiqued Lawler's (1991) proposal that nurses integrate the object body and the lived body in nursing practice. Most nurses talked about being 'holistic' as if they had philosophically moved beyond mechanistic constructions of the body within nursing. It seems to me that nurses have prematurely credited themselves with a paradigm shift that has not yet begun in the Western world. There have been three hundred years of Cartesian constructions of what it might mean to have and be a body. Nursing seems altogether too keen to dismiss this under the rhetorical smoke screen of holism.

Descartes' search for a world that can be treated scientifically, an external world which can be observed, led him to believe that we *have* bodies, but we are *not* bodies (Williams in Magee 1987, p. 86, emphasis added). According to Magee (1987, p. 86), Descartes believed that the body is not part of the 'quintessential me' because he could conceive 'being' without a body. He could not, however, conceive 'being' without conscious awareness. This led him to postulate 'I must irreducibly be thought' (Magee 1987, p. 86).

Williams (in Magee 1987, p. 92) argues that few people now assent to the absolute dualism between the mind and the body and that some distinction between subject and object, knower and known is essential and impossible to do without. However as MR's story will reveal, while people may not assent to the dualism of the body in health care, they have little choice other than to ultimately objectify the body. Williams in (Magee 1987, p. 95), raises Descartes' original questions—What do I know? What can I doubt? What am I? and argues that 'it is a prime philosophical task to arrive at an understanding of oneself, of one's imagination, of one's ideas of what one might be, that can free one from his dualistic model'. I think that this is important because through the stories of MR and others we are now beginning to have a clearer understanding of what 'we are not'.

Lawler (1991, p. 55) argues that although Descartes understood the body in more sophisticated terms than he is usually given credit for, he still nonetheless argued for the existence of both a palpable body and an intangible mind (Scheper-Hughes and Lock 1987, p. 9). According to Scheper-Hughes and Lock (1987, p. 9), Descartes described the soul as being located in the pineal gland where it governed the body. They argue that this separation then preserved 'the soul as the domain of theology' and the body the 'domain of science' which allowed for a 'mechanistic conception of the body and its functions, and a failure to conceptualise a "mindful" causation of somatic states'.

Although men, women and their bodies are fragmented, or reduced to body parts, when the body is theorised through biology and science this fragmentation has more significance to women. Martin (1987, p. 21) argues that women are not only fragmented into body parts through science but they are 'profoundly alienated from science itself'. Laqueur (1990, p. 17) argues that 'science does not simply investigate, but itself constitutes, woman from man'. Martin's (1987) study tells us that women continue to fragment themselves because of the medical language they use to describe their experiences but, as MR's story reveals, there is, as yet, no alternative. It seems that women are often reduced to the position of 'other' to male because of the pervasiveness of male representations of the body in Western society.

ILLNESS STORIES OF THREE MEN

Considering what I have just said about women, it is ironic then that the illness experiences of three people who are men, and two of whom are scientists, Oliver Sacks, Tony Moore and Arthur Frank are examined here. Perhaps these men have been able to write successfully and publish their personal stories because it has been legitimate for them to do so as males and for Sacks and Moore because they are also scientists. Other illness narratives that I read were those of Kleinman (1988), a psychiatrist and an anthropologist, who discusses 'patients' experiences of illness'. While his work is insightful, it differs from the work of Moore, Sacks and Frank in that it is not his own personal story of illness. Frank (1990, p. 140–1) suggests that Kleinman's work offers 'an experience of what it is to be chronically ill in healthist, medicalised America'. Kleinman (1988) most certainly explicates the incompatibility of illness experiences and medical science, but his critique is more helpful for doctors rather than for people who are ill.

Sacks (1984) attributes the incompatibility of the illness experience with medical science to the Cartesian legacy of body and soul. His work, which incorporates what he refers to as neuropsychological and existential phenomena, clearly identifies some of the problems that confronted MR. Sacks (1984, p. 188) argues that the inability of neurology, and thus medicine, to describe his personal illness experience is that 'it excludes mental states, consciousness, because they are "subjective" and "private", and cannot be verified (or validated) in the conventional way'. Sacks (1984, p. 189) believes that ultimately there will be a momentous revolution in medicine, as the 'classical' dualistic, mechanical model that underpins medicine is abandoned for more personal, self referential models. He may be right. However, long before such revolutions are likely to occur, people the world over continue to experience illness silently—their stories never told. And, before any such revolutions, I think we should take the time to understand more fully the incompatibility of the present medical model and the experience of illness itself for both men and women.

I was very grateful that MR had read Oliver Sacks' books *A Leg to Stand On* (1984) and *The Man who Mistook His Wife for a Hat* (1985). This was helpful because she loved his use of narrative and agreed that a 'case study' approach may tell us nothing about her as a person. She particularly liked Sacks' work because he bridges the gulf between what he refers to (in a Cartesian way), as 'the psychical and the physical' and because, Sacks is a scientist using narrative (Sacks 1985, p. x).

Sacks, a physician, had never been a patient before he had an accident on a mountain in Norway. In a bizarre twist of fate Sacks was chased by a bull and, as he was fleeing, he fell and twisted his knee. After suffering a strange paralysis in his leg he describes being alienated from his own leg. Through his personal experiences his work begins to unravel the complexities of illness and the value of narrative in understanding illness experiences. It occurred to me after reading Sacks' work that because he is a doctor he has, somehow, been able to acknowledge the medical narrative that he knows so well and move through that story to find his own. It is a book that I return to time and time again, seduced by the poetics of his writing style and the way he situates himself within the text. The very act of story telling then became important to MR because it situated her and made possible the meanings she could give to her experiences. MR commented that Sacks' stories spoke to her in ways through which she could understand some of her own experiences.

People who have experienced an illness, especially if it is a chronic illness, have difficulty in describing the transition from being well, in a state of healthy existence, to one of being ill. The transition represents something of a crisis in their lives that is ontological in so much as it is about being different. Arthur Frank (1991, p. 13) describes illness as 'the experience of living through the disease' and goes on to say that 'if disease talk measures the body, illness talk tells of the fear and frustration of being inside a body that is breaking down'. In other words there is usually a medical diagnosis which labels the part or parts of the body as a disease and that 'patients' learn to objectify their body by using the language of medical science. Frank (1991) refers to medical language as 'disease talk', as this is language that incorporates the medical treatment. 'Disease talk' is argued by Frank (1991, p. 13) to be designed to make everyone believe that only the disease can be discussed. Exploring this notion further he argues that if you can only discuss the disease there is a gap between what a person feels and that which they feel allowed to say. As Frank's illness progressed he began to feel as if he was in a wide, deep, gap which swallowed his voice and, with it, his story of being ill (Frank 1991, p. 13).

More recently I read Frank's later (1995) work, *The Wounded Story Teller; Body, Illness, and Ethics*. In a similar vein to Sontag (1990), Frank (1995, preface, p. xiii) states 'sooner or later, everyone is a wounded story teller'. He describes how people tell stories through wounded bodies and that 'only a caricature Cartesianism would imagine a head compartmentalised away from the disease, talking about the sick body beneath it' (Frank 1995, p. 2). The attraction to this work is the way that Frank (1995, p. 3) argues that 'ill people need to tell their stories, in order to construct new maps and new perceptions of their relationship to the world'. Frank (1995, p. 5) takes on a postmodern sensibility as he views the modern medical narrative as the story that all stories are judged against as 'true or false, useful or not'.

It was on a Melbourne train, on my way to visit MR, that I finished reading Frank's book. It was a bleak Melbourne day but, as I raised my head to catch the images of stations and backyards rushing by, I was filled with inspiration and hope. I had begun to realise that, like so many nurses, I had listened to illness narratives including MR's in a space that Frank (1995, p. 4) after Borgmann refers to as the 'postmodern divide'. Within this space stories are given new and different meaning and telling a personal story is about reclaiming the space where stories are given primacy (Frank 1995, p. 7). But that was not the only reason I was inspired. I was reflecting on my third-year nursing students and their writings and how I have the pleasure and privilege of reading the most wonderful narrative accounts of their interactions with ill people. Many students are initially confronted by the very idea of exposing something of themselves in their written work. Caught in the story of modernity they are comfortable to be 'other' to themselves.

I spend two semesters with third-year undergraduate students where we work with narrative from a critical perspective. Gradually these students learn to situate themselves and the people they care for in their academic work. As part of the students' assessment they are asked to engage a person who is ill in a conversation that focuses on that person's experience of illness. They learn to recognise the medical narrative as distinct but part of the person's story. This is always difficult because the medical narrative is like a magnet for students who are hungry to become competent clinicians. And people who are ill believe that it is the medical story that they need to tell in order to be heard. Ill people do not usually give voice to their experience of illness in hospital settings unless they are somehow given permission.

Around the wards of the hospital where I work students will be found sitting close to people and taking the time to hear their stories. People's stories of illness are being told and students who will be nurses are learning through these stories. A student told me how she missed the person whose illness narrative she had been listening to after he went home. When I asked her why she simply said 'because I knew him'. I have just finished marking the final work of the year three students. Once again they have included their own stories of the difficulties of listening to an ill person tell their story in a nursing culture that still values 'busyness' and 'professional distance' but they make the comment that the tension it creates is always worthwhile.

Gradually the students begin to understand something of illness through the 'wounded story tellers' (Frank, 1995) that they meet. They write about their experience of listening to these narratives and how they engage as nursing students with people who are ill and they begin to theorise these experiences. Their stories are rich, descriptively powerful narratives—stories about people, illness and nursing. I am always humbled by the experience of coming to know nurses, students and the people they care for through their stories. Nurses, more than any other group of people, develop an understanding of illness through a multitude of stories. As Frank (1995, p. 2) says 'the *personal* issue of telling stories about illness is to give voice to the body, so that the changed body can become once again familiar in these stories'. What nurses do particularly well is to actually hear the body in stories.

Frank (1995, p. 53) poses that 'becoming seriously ill is a call for stories' because of the healing that accompanies telling a personal story and because ill people are asked to tell their story to health workers, friends and family. Using the metaphor of a shipwreck Frank (1995, p. 53) describes some ill people as 'narrative wrecks'. 'The central resource that any story teller depends on is "a sense of temporality" which is suddenly lost, when one becomes ill' (Frank 1995, p. 55). Personal trauma, like illness, can leave a person with a past that is painful to recall, a present that is painful to be in and a sense that there is no future. For MR to think about being fit and healthy in her past was, for her, to feel indescribable grief that would flood over her in waves. The present was to be re-embodied as 'just a head'. But worse than the past or the present was not being able to conceive a future.

Tony Moore (1991) has also written his story of illness following a serious motor vehicle accident and he gives a very descriptive account of living through the language of disease. Moore, a medical practitioner, discusses giving up his body to be 'fixed' and how this caused him to experience being disembodied. He tells us 'when I looked down at my emotional self I saw something foreign. I was distressed by the feeling that the person I had been no longer existed' (Moore 1991, p. 28). Moore had been so concerned with being a mass of broken bones that he accepted being treated as an object because he wanted the staff to focus on his body.

Moore's story is particularly insightful because it exemplifies the notion of 'narrative wreckage' that Frank (1995) refers to. His despair, loneliness and sense of loss was profound but this was the story that he only told himself during the early phase of his illness. The glimpses of the nurses in Moore's story incorporate an actual glimpse of his body. He tells us that one nurse seemed to sense that 'she knew an accident could both smash open a body and break open a life' (Moore 1991, p. 11). Even though he found it difficult to tell his story he describes a time, when he talked with a nurse about his younger life, and how important that was to him (Moore 1991, p. 35).

I was fascinated by Moore's reflections of being a patient and a doctor. He argues that he was 'impotent to act against the disregard [he] occasionally saw expressed by staff towards patients who had neither the will nor the skill to fight for themselves' (Moore 1991, p. 56). Apart from one incident, overall Moore seems to be impressed by the nurses and describes them as 'humane, practical and skilful' (Moore 1991, p. 106). Since he would have spent considerable time with nurses I would have been interested to know some of the stories that led him to describe nurses as humane and skilful. These stories, however, are probably the intimate details of how they managed his body and these are the stories that are rarely told, which is why nursing is so difficult to define as an activity.

Seven years after the accident Moore (1991, p. 142) wrote 'my story attempts to reveal how a *person*, and not just a *body*, recovers following major injury. Where is the therapeutic equivalent of intensive care units for the emotional wounds that leech themselves onto a lacerated body?'. Moore argues that while the technology coupled with physiological efficiency ensured his physical recovery, his spiritual and emotional contusions were often unrevealed, under diagnosed and remained untreated (Moore 1991, pp. 142–3). What Moore had obviously never considered (until much later, if ever) was that 'the human body is a text, a sign, not just a piece of fleshy matter' (Dallery 1989, p. 54).

What Moore's story does not reveal is a critique of the part he played in his own silencing that is reflected in the language through which he chooses to explore his experience. Based on his own understandings, which infer a Cartesian logic, he describes humans as physical, emotional and spiritual. Sacks (1984), Frank (1991), and Moore (1991) theorise their own illness experiences but the significant difference between their experiences and MR's is that they are all powerful, educated men who could bring their stories to expression. Having a diagnosis also enabled these men to be 'legitimately' ill. Initially MR was told that the disabled body she became resulted through a psychosomatic state. What this actually suggests is that 'something' does not exist. Psychosomatic, as an expression, preserves a mind/body duality through implying mental control over a physical reality.

BEING A BODY

According to Sontag (1990, p. 131) the notion of psychosomatic once belonged to psychology, but 'with psychology's new credibility as science, returned to reinfluence medicine', extremely successfully. By locating the cause of MR's illness in her mind, MR was thought to be responsible in some way for her illness. MR has always resisted this position. The alternative MR longed for was to be healthy, as in the absence of disease, or if she could not escape being ill, to be 'really' ill with disease. To be anything else was to be uncertain and uncertainty, as I later discuss, is uncomfortable.

In summary then I have suggested that Cartesian understandings of the world are evident through the discourses of science and medicine and are discursively constructive of ways of being in the world (subjectivity). Within the context of health care there are a 'network of practices, institutions, and technologies that sustain positions of dominance, and subordination' (Bordo 1989, p. 15) that help us to construct the way we are in our bodies. It would seem MR became enmeshed, at times, in collusion with the very forces that alienated her from her own body.

To examine Cartesian understandings of the world of illness is also to examine the relationship between the social and the individual and the various practices and technologies that determine ways of being in the world. While Eagleton (in McLaren 1988, p. 59) makes the point that the body can never be fully represented in discourse, he argues that discourses function to broaden and intensify the body while Silverman (1988 in McLaren 1988, p. 59) argues that 'discursive bodies lean upon and mould real bodies'. McLaren (1988, p. 60) further argues that discourses are enfolded into the very structure of our desire, a process he refers to as the 'politics of enfleshment'. While this is a complex issue, the point he is making is that we do not simply exist within bodies but that we actually are bodies (McLaren 1988, p. 62). It is being a body which is largely ignored in medicine and nursing.

3

READING THE BODY

> *Research approaches inherently reflect our beliefs about the world we live in and want to live in.* (Lather 1991, p. 51)

GETTING STARTED

It was my belief that bodies are largely ignored in nursing scholarship and research that motivated me to write about MR's experiences of being ill. My interest in the life stories of people, however, especially when they are ill began when I first worked as a student nurse. I was seventeen when I began nursing and I was totally unprepared for the experiences I had on the oncology unit where I was sent after preliminary training school. It was my first encounter with an ill person that influenced my decision to continue with nursing. This person was a young woman with cancer. I spent the last week of her life nursing her. It was the conversations that I had with this woman that fixed my interest on the experience of being ill. She told me her story of pain and her suffering in such a way that it became firmly etched upon my memory.

Years later, when I began to teach student nurses it was this story and many more that guided my teaching. These powerful narratives reveal something of the social and material conditions that shape people's lives, and something of what it might mean to be ill. However, all of the stories I had been involved with before MR became ill were of people who had a diagnosis. MR's story unsettled and confronted me because it forced me to think about the ways I had always constructed illness and the body. It had also become clear to me, through my teaching, that initially my understandings of the body were mostly scientific and thus very limited.

I wanted to situate myself in a space to take up the challenge of re-thinking illness, a space where I could tell both MR's story and my story. I especially liked what bell hooks had to say about such spaces. hooks (1990, p. 153) believes she has located herself in the margins of everyday life as a site of resistance and that, as people enter these spaces through suffering and pain, they are drawn to enter such spaces as a critical response to domination. I use the term 'space' because as hooks (1990, p. 152) so eloquently suggests 'spaces can be real and imagined. Spaces can tell stories and unfold histories. Spaces can be interrupted, appropriated, and transformed through artistic and literary practice'. The space where stories can be told and histories unfolded is where I have positioned myself to explore MR's experience of illness—I came to this space through my theorising of our experiences. hooks describes how one can come to such a space:

> Our living depends on our ability to conceptualise alternatives, often impoverished. Theorising about this experience aesthetically, critically is an agenda for radical cultural practice. For me this space of radical openness is a margin—a profound edge. Locating oneself there is difficult yet necessary. It is not a 'safe' place. One is always at risk. One needs a community of resistance. (hooks 1990, p. 149).

SPEAKING OUT

> Yearning is the word that best describes a common psychological state [sic] shared by many of us, cutting across boundaries of race, class, gender, and sexual practice. Specifically, in relation to the post-modernist deconstruction of 'master' narratives, the yearning that wells in the hearts and minds of those whom such narratives have silenced is the longing for critical voice. (hooks 1990, p. 27)

Interestingly the yearning to which hooks (1990) refers not only speaks to my desire to find a critical voice but also highlights the difficulty we all have, even hooks, in moving beyond mind–body dualism. She refers to yearning as 'a common psychological state'. In this study I have found it extremely difficult to escape the binary logic which underpins our world and account for 'difference' and 'subjective' experience 'without avoiding the tension of interrupting the norms of academic writing' (Lather 1991, p. 8). I am referring here to Kramarae and Spender's (1992, p. 1) notion, that the traditional acceptance of what constitutes knowledge, is that knowledge is 'objective, impartial, and neutrally discovered' and that knowledge makers have primarily been men.

Through the process of telling MR's and my story, I position myself precariously beyond the boundaries of what constitutes legitimate knowledge. I believe that it is possible to account for difference and subjective experience through an analysis of the stories that we choose to tell about ourselves. These stories reveal something of the social and material conditions that shape our lives and they can open up the possibilities that there are many 'truths'. According to Weedon (1987, p. 173) 'we have to assume subjectivity in order to make sense of society and ourselves'. Kramarae and Spender (1992, p. 16) argue that the use of stories or biographies is a fertile ground for women to explore as researchers 'because it generates so many issues about the nature of knowledge and authority, about veracity and validity'. I have used a story telling process following Kramarae and Spender, and Weedon as a way for MR and myself to assume subjectivity.

White (1992a) argues that we are shaped and constituted through the process of interpreting experience within the context of stories. Every time a story is told a person is in the process of re-authoring their life and, according to Ricour (1983) in (White 1992a, p. 80), 'there does not seem to be any other mechanism for the structuring of experience that so captures the sense of lived time, or that can adequately represent the sense of lived time'. It is through the story telling process that meaning is given to experience as people determine which aspects of experience they will select for expression in a story (White 1992b, p. 123). White argues that stories are important since they provide structures for living rather than functioning as reflections of life which have no real effects (White 1992b, p. 123).

Although stories provide structures we can live by, I am not suggesting that people live their lives as the stories of their experiences. Kelber (1990, p. 75) argues that 'the art of telling stories has faithfully accompanied the human race from preliterate to post modern times'. However, Kelber (1990, p. 75) referring to White says that 'no one and nothing lives as story, for life itself does not narrate'. Indeed 'stories help to build a world of ontological security and continuity' (Revill 1993, p. 129). De Certeau (in Revill 1993, p. 130) describes stories as 'culturally creative acts' which create the world in which we live.

> This is not a secure world, it only lasts as long as the story is remembered and every time it is retold the world is created anew. But it is a certain world because it is based on the narrative process by which we describe the world to ourselves in our own terms to our own satisfaction, enabling us both to manipulate that world and to move around in it. (de Certeau in Revill 1993, p. 130)

As we manipulate and move around the world through the narrative process many gaps, inconsistencies, and contradictions emerge as our stories unfold. White (1992b, p. 125), asserts this activity is important since it provokes people into 'meaning making' which involves making unique sense out of their lives as they try to resolve some of the gaps and inconsistencies. He also argues that our lives are constituted through a process of meaning making through story telling as we live and then re-tell the story of our experiences, in contrast to the view that the experiences or the 'lived' experiences are reality there to be uncovered or found (White 1992b, p. 125). The process of re-telling a story can open up spaces and possibilities for alternative stories to emerge. People can become free to explore an alternative story when they can separate themselves from the dominant or 'totalising' stories that constitute their lives (White 1992b, p. 127). Totalising stories are those grand narratives such as the Cartesian narrative of the mind and the body.

GRAND TOTALISING STORIES

One way of becoming aware of the implications totalising stories have on people and their lives is to allow a story to emerge and stand by itself without it having to be compared to a normative structure. Lyotard (1984) has referred to the overarching philosophies of history as 'grand and totalising narratives' that attempt to speak for all of human kind all of the time. It is through these grand narratives that we have come to engage with notions of the normal body. Parry (1991, p. 40) argues most convincingly that 'the very notion of the norm as applied to differences between people, the problems that arise, and of the difficulties in embracing those differences, is the source of the pathologising tendency'.

MR's story reveals that without a diagnosis she could not and indeed has not found a way to have her experiences validated, not only by medicine, but also by nursing and people in general. MR was, in a sense, silenced by the power of the medical narrative. Medicine from this vantage point has this power because 'its voice [is] sanctified by its sacred text and its story objectified as history' (Parry 1991, p. 40). Casey (in De Concini 1990, p. 46) suggests that 'narrative remembering', or a person's ability to tell their story, is crucial to how people sustain an identity 'over time as continuously the same person'. This suggests that stories are constitutive of our lives rather than the belief that experience is the reality.

STORIES AS BEING CONSTITUTIVE OF OUR LIVES

My interest in story telling is also about me as a woman valuing the lived experiences of other women that come to expression through their stories (Campbell and Bunting 1991, p. 7; Smith and Watson 1992; Gluck and Patai 1991). I believe that 'the deafening silence of women's voice and experience in Western culture and history' discussed by Dallery (1989, p. 53) is one of the main imperatives that should guide women engaged in scholarship and research. According to Webster-Barbre et al. (1989, p. 4) 'Listening to women's voices, studying women's writings, and learning from women's experiences have been crucial to the feminist reconstruction of our understanding of the world'. Assuming 'men have constructed the prevailing theories, written history, and set values that have become the guiding principles for men and women alike' this is a difficult and contentious issue for female scholars (Belenky et al. 1986, pp. 5–6). The way that MR and I assume the personal in the initial study and in our book represents what is a difficult journey for women in the academy who are generating knowledge, and, at the same time, coming to a critical voice.

I have argued so far that our lives can be shaped and understood through narratives (Cohler 1982) and the very act of story telling can illuminate, transform and reveal how a person's life can be understood (Sandelowski 1991). However, Kelber (1990, p. 75) argues that we do not usually give critical attention to our narrative impulses and performances and that, which we mostly take for granted, obviously eludes our full attention.

Nurses are immersed in the stories of others, yet Sandelowski (1991, p. 162) argues they have not explored directly the storied nature of human interpretation and placed it at the centre of their scholarship and research. Nurses have certainly explored the 'lived experiences' of people through phenomenology, but they have not worked with stories and narratives within a more critical framework. Dickson (1990, p. 60) suggests that when nurses entered the academic field they began to emulate other scholars and primarily based their studies on the established scientific way of knowing. The scientific research tradition has masked the knowledge nursing generates since it does not provide a framework to theorise the experiences of people, including nurses themselves. As 'other' to medicine, nurses have been searching for a space from which to speak. The marginality and oppression embodied in nurses' experiences has silenced their stories and, simultaneously, those of the people they care for. Furthermore because nursing is primarily an oral culture (Street 1992b), the stories of nursing are not usually captured in text. In fact most nurses resist any written practices because, in general, they are not actively attempting to change their taken for granted ways of being.

The enormous resistance for nurses not to participate in any written practices is discussed by Street (1992a). She found that clinical nurses argue their interests lie in providing quality care to 'patients', not in writing which is seen as a waste of time for the 'busy nurse' (Street 1992a, p. 19). Yet we know that nurses have intimate contact with people and that primarily nursing is an oral culture of telling stories. Spreen Parker (1990) tells us that she has never met a nurse who does not have a story to tell because the art of story telling is practised in almost every facet of nursing. Spreen Parker (1990, p. 39) argues that to maintain what she calls 'personal integrity', or what I understand as confidentiality, most nurses' stories have been silenced and rendered unspeakable. Hays (1989, p. 202), in Foucauldian tradition, argues that nurses have been silenced because they are constrained in practice by 'the fellowship of discourse'. Who should speak and what should be said is strictly regulated within a closed community. The stories that nurses tell stay within the oral culture of nursing.

Walker (1995) discusses the bureaucratic and clinical discourses that inform nursing and describes the tension in nursing between the former, which values the written, and the latter which values the spoken. He says that these discourses have remained largely untheorised and that this is why such contradictions continue to shape nursing culture (Walker 1995). Walker (1995, p. 161) proposes that '. . . nurses' sense of themselves has been locked into modes of desire (after McLaren 1988) in which the "other" is always white, male and endowed with certain knowledges; knowledges which inscribe authority, influence and privilege on the bodies of those who claim to possess them'. A person's sense of self is captive to certain knowledges and dominant 'regimes of truth' (Foucault 1980) which can be contested, challenged and deconstructed through the telling of narratives. Deconstructing authority is not to do away with it. Rather, it is to see how authority is constituted and constituting of our lives (Lather 1991, p. 144).

THE POLITICS OF WRITING THE SELF AND OTHERS

MR and I had shared many stories together as friends but, when I formalised our relationship as co-researchers for the study and we began to tape the narratives for transcription, MR became enthusiastic to the point that she seemed driven. The study formalised a commitment from both of us to indulge in story telling. It was quite poignant that without this process in place we may have never heard each other's stories in such a meaningful way. MR told me that telling her story in this way had been therapeutic for her. Perhaps this was because MR found a space to give voice to the privilege of speaking (Walker 1993, p. 7).

Later when we had the flexibility to move beyond the research to writing this book we found that we still followed some of the structures we had used for the research. That is we always went back over the stories (re-storying) which enabled us to add a rich depth of understanding that we both shared. This was to be an exciting time because MR with her voice-activated computer was now able to produce her own text. She theorised another layer around the work that I had submitted as a study then I went to Melbourne so that we could engage in a story telling process face to face. I then dealt with the process of weaving yet another story (mine) into the text again. Then with the assistance of e-mail we continued to ask each other questions. I would have to say that I found this particularly difficult because it forced me to work with the inevitable tension of whose voice was privileged.

Walker (1993, p. 235) argues that when theorists and participants in research jostle for space there are many voices to privilege and this creates a tension for the researcher. Reflecting on his doctoral study, Walker (1993, p. 236), makes the point that 'one voice is necessarily privileged over the others' and in his study it was his because he had a question to answer. Although we have not escaped this tension, I believe that we have minimised it through a process of 'joint story telling' (after Lumby 1992) so that 'our individual reflections and our joint conversations formed the foundation of our meanings and of our journey together' (Lumby 1992, p. 116).

I believe that the way I approached the telling of both MR's and my stories in the initial study 'disrupts' the received norms in research by a certain 'textual self-consciousness' referred to by Lather (1991, p. 150) after van Manen. This book has allowed us to explore this notion further in that MR and I hope to critique the taken for granted understandings of what it means to be ill in the 1990s.

> Disallowing claims to certainty, totality and Archimedean standpoints outside of flux and human interest, it is to tell a 'story that retrieves inquiry as a "way" that is always already beginning, always already "on the way"', a different story 'that makes a critical difference not only at the site of thought but also at the site of sociocultural praxis'. (Spanos in Lather 1991, p. 151)

THE MEETING OF FRIENDS

When I began the study it had been my intention to meet with MR every week in her home but we met every night in the first week, several hours at a time. We both enjoyed this time and the intensity and frequency seemed important. We chose evenings when MR would be in bed after the evening nurse had visited. Initially we experienced an urgency to tell our stories and tried to tell them using a chronological sequence of events. It was this linear sequence of events that allowed us to move into our stories. Kermode (in Sandelowski 1991, p. 163) suggests 'the mind is put to rest by the illusion of sequence and order, the appearance of causality and the look of necessity'. As MR and I became more comfortable with the whole process our story telling style seemed to change. Although our stories eventually became non-linear, there was always sequence which De Concini (1990, p. 115) argues is important, because in memory there has to be sequence for experience to be coherent.

Initially we were both somewhat nervous having moved from being friends to being friends and doing research. Almost as soon as our individual stories merged into conversation MR raised the issue that it appeared our rememberings for the same period of time we shared were different. These differences were discussed at some length. We were beginning to discover, as Weedon (1987, p. 79) suggests, 'what an event means to an individual depends on the ways of interpreting the world, on the discourses available to her at any particular moment'. Our beginning conversations exposed the liberal humanistic assumptions that we both subscribed to concerning 'the transparency of language and the fixity of subjectivity' (Weedon 1987, p. 83). We were analysing the events as we both remembered them to decide on the 'truth'. At this time MR and I assumed that there must be some certainty and that there was indeed a truth to *confirm our* experiences. From these conversations, MR and I found that our experiences were always 'open to contradictory and conflicting interpretation', since the plurality of language makes fixing meaning near impossible (Weedon 1987, p. 85).

MR was particularly interested in story telling as a method because, as a scientist and a researcher, she wondered if this was 'real' research and asked me questions about rigour, reliability, validity and so on. Initially she saw her story as a 'medical case history' and this affected the way she chose to talk about her experience. I believe that a case study can be a form of narrative, but is usually not a story telling style that captures people's experiences. I was not comfortable with a case study approach because, as Benner (1991, p. 16) argues, 'stories—as opposed to case studies or analytic reports—engage persons in a learning dialogue with their own historical understanding and personal knowledge'.

It seemed MR was more familiar and comfortable with 'all of those literary devices that separate authors from their text' such as writing in the third person (Sandelowski 1991, p. 161). We discussed how it was only more recently, undertaking a postgraduate degree, that I had been taught by academics to situate the self in my work (Benhabib 1992; Walker 1994c). Along with many of the arguments that Webb (1992) puts forward supporting writing in the first person in academic work, I now avoid the methodological tension of writing in such a way that I become 'other' to myself. Initially, the way I used the 'I' was difficult for MR because her scientific training had taught her to make sure she was always 'other' to herself. She would have achieved this through the separation of method, results and interpretation in her own scientific work (Sandelowski 1991, p. 161). This approach that scientists use is considered to be 'anti-narrative' (Sandelowski 1991, p. 161). These conversations became important for MR and me in so much as they became spaces for us to become critical in our intent and to be comfortable with uncertainty.

REFLECTIONS ON NARRATIVE AS A METHOD

As in all writing the politics and ethics of deciding to tell a particular story is of concern. In this book (after Lather 1993), I was concerned with the issues of how to tell a story that MR and I share and how I would take the 'crisis of representation' into account (Lather 1991, pp. 21–5). Walker (1994a, p. 46) argues that this crisis not only involves how to represent the voices of others, but also the voices of the theorists that are drawn upon to theorise the story. It is a struggle that he described as the difficulty of speaking for oneself and others.

I have wrestled with all of the uncertainties involved in how to represent myself and others in this work. According to Probyn (1993, p. 4) 'embodying a care of self in speech and in writing' is a necessity 'to construct ways of thinking marked by "me" but that do not efface actively or through omission the ways in which "she" may see differently'. As I have clearly placed myself in the text the tension, for me, became one of constantly making sure I have not spoken for MR when she could speak for herself, and that I try to avoid obscuring her voice with mine. I have tried to emphasise the historical conditions involved in speaking, in this book, through a critical use of the self (Probyn 1993, p. 28). Moreover my representations of MR or myself are not innocent; as they always presuppose particular modes of understanding of which we may or may not be conscious at their moment of representation.

To tell this story I have worked with the tension of both MR and myself having many stories to tell. There has been a necessary intersection of our stories that we had to became comfortable with to enable another story to be told. Probyn (1993, p. 171) addresses this problem theoretically by suggesting 'because of the material conditions of our selves we cannot indulge in the fantasy of dialogism wherein "you" can be "me" and "I" you. "I" am not "she" but articulating a working image of the self may allow for a movement of empathy between us'.

The theoretical considerations in situating the self are important to consider since the telling of this story is not a process of self indulgent affirmation of our experiences (Probyn 1993, p. 30). Narrative can be a research technology that 'contests those "received" understandings of what constitutes good research' (Walker 1995, p. 157). In this book I have appropriated narrative as a means to explore and speak the body through the text (Probyn 1993, pp. 30–1). Probyn (1993) does this especially well by weaving her narrative rememberings of living with anorexia, with dense theoretical arguments on situating the self as a textual strategy.

THE POLITICS OF MORALITY

The difficult, and perhaps insuperable, problem in situating MR and I in this text, is addressed by Sacks (1990) in his work, *Awakenings*. He asks, how does one 'convey detailed information without betraying professional and personal confidence', and still 'preserve what is important'? (Sacks 1990, preface). How ethical is it to tell this story—whose is it—and whose interests does it serve? I feel I need to make explicit some of the ethical issues that are the history of this book.

MR and I had a unique opportunity to work as co-researchers not only because of our friendship but also because of our similar intellectual histories. MR was familiar with universities and the nature of tertiary study. She has a Bachelor of Science with Honours and after she became ill had to convert her PhD to be awarded a Master of Science. With this background she was very aware of ethical considerations in research and the implications of possibly being identified in the initial study. The benefits for MR were varied and complex at that time. She argued that it was therapeutic and cathartic to tell her story and that a critique of her illness experience was insightful for her because it helped her come to terms with her illness.

Our friendship was a critical ethical issue because I have had to consider such issues as: have either of us taken advantage of our friendship unfairly; would this journey affect our friendship detrimentally; did MR feel as a friend, that she could withdraw from the process if she wanted to; could I; would she regret the telling of her story? These questions largely remain but interestingly when the study was completed MR hated being anonymous. She wanted to have the opportunity to be MR in the text and this book allows her to be visible.

4

THE BODY AS TEXT

BODY OF SCIENCE

I have argued that the friendship MR and I both share has been a critical issue in the writing of this book. The stories of our friendship continue as MR's story of becoming ill is explored further. The critical conversations that we had around the stories deepened our understandings of MR's illness experiences. We continued our journey as friends and as two people writing a book. The complexity of juxtaposing the more formal process that began with the study, and the continuing narrative of our friendship, is evident by the way I have necessarily assumed the position of friend, theorist and self in the text. MR has a story to tell and indeed, so do I. My own narrative rememberings are interwoven within the analysis and, as I have said previously, are problematic at times because, sometimes they are me, sometimes MR, and sometimes 'other' to both of us.

This chapter is called 'The Body as Text' and was so named because of the profound discomfort I began to feel as MR started to tell her story. Her story began to expose how Cartesian understandings of the body have so dramatically shaped but at the same time concealed her story and thus her experiences. The rich descriptive stories of MR's experiences, the tragic story of her despair, loneliness and grief can only be glimpsed beneath the text. The stories that I, and perhaps you, would expect to hear and read are, somehow, seemingly trapped within MR's body and it is her 'body as text' that tells that story. In this chapter MR's body becomes her most 'intimate' yet at the same time 'alienating possession' (Diprose 1991, p. 67). The stories are a harsh reminder of the exclusion of 'consciousness' and 'being' from medical science. Diprose (1991, pp. 67–8) explains this by stating that 'we can only "dwell" in a world, encounter objects within it and be encountered as an object (say, by science) if we are constituted by a set of relations with which we are, thereby, familiar'.

The Cartesian legacy that dominates the set of relations that constitutes 'being' for most people has cast the experiences of embodiment into an abyss of silence. Harth (1992, p. 9) argues this point by proposing that 'Cartesian rationalism' opened a 'discursive trap' with which women have struggled for centuries. Furthermore Harth (1992, p. 6) argues that it is the Cartesian legacy which has 'contributed heavily to a totalising rational discourse of abstract universality and objectivity from which women by the historical contingencies of their gender became excluded'. I have emphasised this because MR has struggled with exclusions at many levels—professionally as a female scientist and personally as an ill woman without a diagnosis.

BEING BURIED ALIVE IN OUR CULTURE

In a similar vein Whitford suggests that 'a danger of our times is that the knower has become split off from the embodied and social subject' (Whitford 1991, p. 149). She argues that this split is far more significant for women because 'if women are cut off from their own becoming, then they are "buried alive" in our culture' (Whitford 1991, p. 149). This statement is a poignant suggestion of why MR's experiences of being ill are only to be glimpsed beneath the text; in other words, I am suggesting that MR is buried alive resulting from the process of the objectification of her body as a woman (see also Diprose 1994) and from not having a diagnosis. The enigma of the body is captured by this process as MR, in her desperate attempt to 'be a body', 'some body', ultimately becomes 'no body', just a head.

Before MR was to describe herself as abandoned she travelled a journey that many people who have experienced illness may recognise. This is the traditional journey of becoming a Cartesian body, a body for investigation by science. Residing in the 'kingdom of the sick', MR lost more and more sense of her self and eventually constructed her 'being', as a head. As MR objectifies her own body as a body of science she appears to be lost or buried alive within this chapter. This is how MR introduced herself through her narrative rememberings, before she moves through her story to her experiences of being ill. MR chooses to introduce herself in the historical present (Probyn 1993, p. 108).

A WOMAN OF SCIENCE

MR: Where in your life do you start—when you can say that things are relevant to how you are now? That's difficult isn't it. I guess for me, I don't really think I became a person until I left home, went to Uni, was free to do what I wanted without my parents. So I don't think I became MR until I went to Uni. I was seventeen then. I have always been an extremely independent spirit but first felt free to be the real me at that time. My dad was married before so I've got a half brother and a sister and I had a brother who died in a motor bike accident in 1984; my mother died in 1989. I felt the loss of my mother in particular as we were also close friends and kindred spirits. My respect for my mother's intelligence, integrity and compassion was, and is, boundless.

My mother's death was really bad timing because I had just completed my honours in science and the graduation was the next day. Because I was removed from it, I think it took a while for it to sink in. After my mother's funeral I went back to uni to pursue my PhD. I really enjoyed research because it was interesting to find out things that no-one else had ever found out before. It had a certain amount of tedium involved in it because you do repetitive things, obviously, in scientific research, to get results. If you are doing quantitative research you've got to do a certain number of experiments to get your answers. I just found it really interesting—I enjoyed the work. I used to spend seven days a week on it. I just loved it. But I also wanted to be an academic because that was a way I knew I could be in a university system with a permanent job and also be able to do independent research.

Besides research my second love was sport and I loved skiing . . . snow skiing. I used to do it at every opportunity in the winter. We used to pop up to Mount Buller and we always had our annual pilgrimage to Falls Creek. I used to love skiing. I also played hockey for my University—I loved hockey. I was also getting into triathlons. I was training . . . doing heaps of running, or riding my bike everywhere; any time when I wasn't teaching or doing research I was training. So I had a pretty active full life, I was very happy then. It was a big decision to move interstate to a new job.

That is how I met you (Denise). The first time we met it was to discuss possible changes to the science course being taught to nursing students. We were both on a committee and once we came together we found we had some pretty common goals. You and I were new staff members and there were a lot of pre-existing prejudices between nursing and science, a lot of old hostility between nursing and science, so it was a difficult thing we were doing. Basically we helped develop and write a new curriculum. We pioneered it. It was actually a good time—it was a watershed, wasn't it? It was a good time to be involved, and I feel quite proud of what we achieved. I'm quite sort of sad that I am not a part of that any more. I think we developed a friendship as co-conspirators. We had goals for nursing.

Do you remember I broke my ankle and had to have plaster on it for three months after walking around on it for ages after it was broken? But then after I got my plaster off I was really unfit and fat and I needed to indulge in some exercise. I think that's how we got started. I think you and I discussed that we both shared a common desire to get thinner. We started off walking almost immediately when I got out of plaster; we actually ended up doing some running. It was great. It was on one of our walks that I had an asthma attack. I have got a strong family history of asthma, but was not diagnosed as having asthma until the age of twenty. I must admit that I have been a very non-compliant asthmatic, because I didn't really believe in the medication. I do know, though, that asthma is a very insidious disease, in that you don't realise the damage you are doing by not treating it. Ultimately I ended up in ICU with asthma after one of our walks—only I was too sick to remember an awful lot of what was going on at that time.

From MR's story it becomes clear just how important being a scientist was to her as she tells us how she valued her life as a scientist. However, as a female scientist in the academy there were many issues concerning the 'structural investments and patriarchal commitments in science' that undoubtedly affected her career (Grosz and de Lepervanche 1988, p. 5). It is the exclusion of women in science that has contributed to gender being constitutively operative in science (Keller, 1985). Keller (1989, p. 42) argues that this exclusion of women, and that which is known as feminine, 'has been historically constitutive of a particular definition of science—as incontrovertibly objective, universal, impersonal—and masculine: a definition that serves simultaneously to demarcate masculine from feminine and scientists from non-scientists—even good science from bad'.

Namenwirth (1986, p. 24) takes this point further by saying there is an 'excessive and destructive level of competition' in academic science. I recall that MR was faced with this tension at work. Namenwirth (1986, p. 23) argues that if women in science display competitive type behaviours it would invite criticism and, conversely, if they behave as women are expected, that is supportive and docile, they are not seen as pursuing their careers with the 'appropriate level of vigour and drive' to be 'good' scientists.

An important part of MR's background is nutrition and this worked against her because, according to Hubbard (1990, p. 44), women are said to be connected to this branch of science because of its links to home economics. It must have been extremely difficult for MR to belong in the world of science, but it was a world where she carved out for herself a life that she passionately embraced. This high level of tension is important, when considering MR's history as a female scientist, because these same tensions surface and trouble MR as she assumes the role of a sick patient.

In MR's story we hear that she was a very active person. She tells us about being involved in a variety of sports. She only touches on the issue of asthma briefly and describes herself as non-compliant by resisting medications, despite knowing that asthma is an insidious disease. MR gives the impression, from this story, that she is not someone familiar with being ill. She was a fit, active person living a full life at the time she entered the hospital as a 'patient'. I think this is an important point since MR was probably thrust or hurled into being ill rather than entering this state gradually. Both of our stories reveal the way MR was thrust into being ill by the way she was walking with me one minute and then on her way to ICU within an hour.

A JOURNEY THROUGH INTENSIVE CARE: A SPACE OF PRIVILEGES

MR: Talking and writing about my experiences in ICU is still extremely difficult and painful. I am still haunted by my time in ICU and my psychiatrist says, that as a result of that time, I have Post Traumatic Stress Disorder. It is as if it was just filmed yesterday and the video player is never far from my consciousness. My dreams were filled with ventilators, alarms sounding, people dying, pain and fear and me struggling for every breath. I believe that something went catastrophically wrong with my body in ICU. I don't remember much about casualty but when I first became aware I was in ICU my body was covered with a bewildering array of monitors, intravenous lines and other tubes. I was familiar with the tubes but not like this. I think I looked at my body and thought does that belong to me? On day two I got worse and my oxygen saturations plummeted and my respiration rate dropped off. I had to have adrenalin nebs and all of that stuff . . . anyway I can remember I thought I was going to die. I remember sitting; you know, the best position is to sit up and over, leaning over. I was sitting in that position and the physio was sitting behind me and she had her arms around my diaphragm (you know, around the side of me) and she was saying, 'Come on, you can breathe'. And I remember I was breathing something like two times a minute—and I just couldn't breathe. I guess they called the doctors in, they were all around staring at me; one of them told me I couldn't breathe for myself and they were going to have to put me on a ventilator . . . that's all I remember. But I remember the physio sitting behind me, and then I don't remember anything else until I had a sore throat. It was awful having a great big tube being pulled out . . . it was foul—this big thing coming out of your mouth. Anyway, after I came off the ventilator I was very weak; I sort of couldn't move properly or swallow.

MR had been ventilated for a few days until she could breathe again independently. I remember the day I went to see her after she had come off the ventilator. ICU was not a friendly place to visit. I stood outside some doors, pressed a button and spoke to an anonymous nurse who, after some time, let me in. I was not comfortable visiting MR in ICU. I found it to be an alienating environment. I will always remember seeing MR lying limp in a bed. As I sat down beside her tears rolled down her cheeks and she held my hand. I remember this incident because it was one of the few times I had ever seen MR cry—she rarely touched people—they usually touched her. She had looked absolutely exhausted from being ventilated and sedated.

MR: I vaguely remember Denise coming in to see me and feeling the comfort of her holding my hand. When my condition had become more serious none of my friends could come in and see me. This created confusion outside because no-one would tell anyone what was going on. Inside hospital connections enabled them to find out. I'm not sure how Denise had been able to see me, but I'm glad she did.

I did not even stop to consider whether I could visit MR, I just did.

MR: I remember they watched me all of the time in ICU and I had cardiac and respiratory monitors on which went off all of the time. I felt really weak, and I felt really tired. I wasn't really getting any better but I thought they would find out what was wrong with me, so I wanted them to test everything. It's hard to explain how I felt, I just felt really unwell and the nurses started to worry that I was very flaccid—they kept a very close eye on me.

MR makes it clear that she wanted the medical staff to test everything. She was prepared to let the doctors and nurses objectify her body, to carry out investigations 'on' her. Foucault's (1977) analysis of the body as an object and target of power in his work *Discipline and Punish* helps make sense of this. Foucault (1977, p. 136) makes reference to the army, school and hospital, as institutions that control or correct the operations of the body. He argues that as the human body enters spaces such as those set aside for 'patients' in a hospital, it enters 'a machinery of power that explores it, breaks it down and rearranges it' (Foucault 1977, p. 138). MR had entered such a space and she expected and was indeed comfortable with her body being broken down and rearranged.

In hospitals, through the disciplines and practices of medicine and nursing, there is a 'mechanics of power' in play that through 'a policy of coersions that act upon the body', then produces 'subjected and practiced bodies, "docile" bodies' (Foucault 1977, p. 138). MR, in the role of a patient, allows this 'mechanics of power' to take place because, in the same way as inmates in prison or children in schools are, she is compromised. The notion of docility that results from being compromised allows MR's body to be analysed and manipulated at the same time. This process is far more obvious in ICU because of the seriousness of peoples' illnesses and because there is more of an expectation to leave all of the decision making to the 'experts'. Walker takes this point further and argues that ICU is, in fact, a place where 'science has become

institutionalised as *power* and the 'will to truth' is a key dimension of that historical process' (Barrett 1991 in Walker 1993, p. 134).
ICU in this sense becomes a panoptic space. By this I mean that the panopticon architectural design, described and theorised by Foucault (1977) was evident in this particular ICU. Foucault discusses the Panopticon as a mechanism of surveillance of inmates in the prison system (Foucault 1977, p. 201). He claims that by organising people in such a way, observation or surveillance of many people can take place at one time. It can, he argues, 'induce in the inmate, a state of conscious and permanent visibility that assures the automatic functioning of power' (Foucault 1977, p. 201). In the centre of ICU was a raised platform from where doctors and nurses could see all of the patients. MR was able to say that the nursing staff were able to keep a close eye on her partly by way of this architecture.

Under the inspecting gaze of the doctors and nurses I felt most uncomfortable being watched when I visited MR in ICU. As Foucault has argued 'the panopticon is a marvellous machine that, whatever use one may wish to put it to, produces homogeneous effects of power', and this is what I was experiencing (Foucault 1977, p. 202). Power in ICU is not held by anyone in particular but there are positions of dominance because not everyone in the ICU space are equal. Rather for MR it was the way she was positioned in ICU that is relevant here (Bordo 1993, p. 191). Because of the hierarchical nature of hospitals, the nurses and the doctors were able to exercise a certain power through the maintenance and surveillance of MR's body.

MR: The nurses would speak to the doctors about me when they were really worried, which was good because they didn't do that on the ward. They knew I had this strange feeling of being weak, if I moved around in the bed I would flop over to the side and I couldn't get back. When the specialist came the nurse told the doctor what was going on. You (Denise) were there when she did that.

I remember the ward round to which MR refers. The specialist stood at the end of the bed, and it was the nurse who gave him a 'handover'. They had a conversation about MR's medical status at the end of her bed. The nurse carefully threaded a little of 'Oh, and MR is still very weak and we (the nurses) are concerned with how little she can move'. The doctor then turned his gaze towards

MR. He moved in closer to her. This was an interesting use of geographical space, with the nurse, a woman and smaller than the doctor (a male) gazing up at the doctor away from MR the patient. Then the nurse stood aside as the doctor gazed down at MR, another woman, smaller than him and horizontal in bed. Foucault (in Bordo 1993, p. 191) argues:

> There is no need for arms, physical violence, material constraints. Just a gaze. An inspecting gaze, a gaze which each individual under its weight will end by interiorising to the point that he [sic] is his own overseer, each individual thus exercising this surveillance, over and against himself.

MR had been grateful that the nurse had told the doctor that they were worried about her being weak which suggests that she was either not prepared to mention this herself or that she knew the doctor would take more notice of the nurse than her. Despite this, however, the nurse returned to MR saying that the doctors had decided that she could go back to the ward because her breathing was so much better now. There was no mention of the muscle weakness by the doctor at this time.

MR: They decided to take me back to the ward, but really I was no better; worse, in fact. I was a bit scared to go to sleep after being in ICU in case I stopped breathing. It took me months to get over that, because who would know if I stopped breathing at night on the ward? I didn't understand what was going on; at this point, I still thought I had asthma and that's what it was, and I didn't really understand.

MR was scared to leave ICU because as a patient and a scientist she most certainly saw ICU as a space of privileges where she had access to the best and most sophisticated technology available, medical specialists and 'intelligent' nurses. MR tells us that the ICU nurses were worried about her. She has afforded these nurses with the intelligence *to worry* which she does not do with the nurses on the ward. The ICU nurses could be seen as having a privileged position, because they work closely with doctors and therefore science and 'truth'. MR had come to trust the ICU nurses over the ward nurses because of their positioning to the doctors and science.

MR was scared on the ward because she was no longer being monitored technologically and the nurses and doctors were less visible. Being under surveillance in ICU had meant placing her body in the care of others and she was relying on the 'experts'. Leder (1984, p. 35) argues that in doing this, 'there is an ironical fulfilment of Cartesian dualism—a mind (namely, that of the doctor) runs a passive and extrinsic body (that of the "patient")'. The objectification of MR's body achieved through a 'mechanics of power' in ICU is different on the ward where the docility of her body is assured rather more subtly through other disciplinary practices and codes of behaviour (Foucault 1977, p. 137). MR's remarks, about who would know if she stopped breathing on the ward, indicate how she felt the 'gaze' was somewhat minimised on the ward in comparison to ICU.

THE BODY DETECTIVE

The most worrying feature of MR's experiences at this time was the lack of concern over her continuing muscle weakness. The transition back to the ward without any explanation about this was extremely difficult for her and she began to struggle to locate this 'thing' with no name herself. MR had been led to believe that perhaps her asthma and muscle weakness were related since they had never been separated as different problems. This belief probably kept her remarkably calm as the obedient patient—patiently waiting to get better, even though she repeatedly was saying she was actually getting worse.

MR: So there I was on the ward getting worse: I could not initiate movements with my arms and legs, or sustain the movement and carry it through to a completed action; swallowing was the same where the food would get stuck in my throat, and I coughed and spluttered. I started to get the breathing difficulty back and one day I was trying to move in the bed and I fell out onto the floor. They were worried again so took me back to ICU because my blood gases had deteriorated again. This time while I was in ICU, I thought about the pathways; the pneumotaxic centre and the relationship between that and the respiratory centre and, you know, it didn't make sense. I must admit I did try and analyse; like, I always wanted to know what my blood pressure was, and what everything was. I was very interested in that side of things, but I didn't understand what was going on. I remember it was really hard to move around in the bed, trying to move and sort of flopping over the side. I wanted to get out of there this time because people were so sick and the lady in the bed next to me had the ventilator turned off and her family were crying around her bed. It was awful. I said to the doctor 'Get me out of here, get me back to the ward'.

Once again we hear MR flag the point that she only went back to ICU because of her blood gases (her lungs) and her concerns about being unusually weak are still being ignored. Her faith in the doctors came into question and momentarily MR describes moving out of the patient role as she stood back from herself trying to understand her body as a scientist might. She puts herself into the uncomfortable position of investigating her own body. MR acknowledges this tension by saying that it is not acceptable for patients to analyse themselves scientifically. She was not prepared to be the passive patient, because the doctors had so far let her down. Their investigations had not acknowledged that asthma was far from being a diagnosis that encompassed all of the symptoms that she was experiencing. Indeed, they had not seemed to have listened to, or have heard, her concerns about the changes in her body. In these moments of resistance, MR was able to bring to expression how on one level she was the 'docile body' biologically disempowered, and how on another level she was prepared to contest this.

This is a moment of resistance in as much as MR objectifies herself. She has spoken of feeling guilty because she dared to suppose that she had the right or authority to think about her body scientifically. The only person in a hospital who claims this space is the undisputed voice of authority, the doctor, who speaks with the voice of science. This voice is legitimate as opposed to the voice of the patient who possesses only local and untrained knowledges and skills (Foucault 1980). Often the voice of the doctor diminishes and minimises the voice of the patient to the point that it is silenced.

Perhaps MR as a scientist was not afraid to claim back some of the power that silences anyone 'other' than the doctor. Since the question of her muscle weakness was being ignored she began to ask questions at every opportunity of anyone who came into contact with her. The nurses, physiotherapists, and the pharmacists all echoed the same reply: *'You will have to ask your doctor'*. This is yet another example of MR's need to have a conversation about herself being denied to her. Each one of these qualified people would be unlikely to engage in talking to MR about her illness because she had not got a diagnosis. These people disqualify their own knowledges by being as silent as the patient. Foucault (1980, p. 82) suggests that this happens because of the subjugation of knowledge, 'a whole set of knowledges that have been disqualified as inadequate to their task or insufficiently elaborated: naive knowledges, located low down on the hierarchy, beneath the level of cognition or scientificity'. I am arguing then that the silences that became a major part of MR's experiences are partly because of the power/knowledge relations Foucault (1980) refers to.

MR: As my asthma improved my muscle weakness got worse and the nurses moved me into a room with three really sick women. The doctors didn't come to see me as much, and I had a lot of time to think about what might be happening to me. That was when I used to want to read my medical history to check my results because no one seemed worried about how weak I was getting. I thought they must be missing something. Surely something would show up.

MR became concerned that the doctors may have overlooked some vital clues in her 'case' so she began to take a keen interest in what was, and what was not, being done to her. When I visited her, she would talk very quietly to me, in case the other women in the ward heard. The screens were always drawn, and MR would whisper to me her biochemistry results, her blood pressure readings, and all of the other data that she had 'secretly' collected. She would ask me to get her charts off the end of the bed and hold them up for her to read. I began to feel guilty because I was complicit in the secrecy that began to shroud MR's investigations. Moreover, I was worried that the nurses would see or hear me and, despite all the rhetoric regarding advocacy and rights of patients, to read one's own medical charts is transgressing a taken-for-granted boundary.

With MR's focus now decidedly on her biological body she only discussed herself mechanistically—reducing her body to a network of systems, examining it system by system. She reminded me of a detective, a body detective, searching for clues as to the cause of her illness. The problem was she was not officially recognised as being assigned to the case so she had become secretive, concealing her intention from the official detectives, the doctors.

MR: I was worried because I still couldn't breathe properly, and I couldn't swallow. I just couldn't. I had to make myself breathe.

The ladies in my room all had cancer and they kept talking about their illnesses. I just listened to them but couldn't really talk about what was happening to me. Day after day I got sicker. No-one knew what was wrong with me and eventually they moved me to a single room again. I thought it was because they thought they might catch something from me.

Denise: Did they say that?

MR: No.

Denise: But you had the feeling that they thought you were contagious?

MR: Yes . . . or they were scared. I remember some of the nurses not wanting to nurse me because when I ate, I got mucous plugs stuck in my throat, and it was scary; they were frightened I was going to 'cark' it on them—not that they said so.

Denise: How did you know that?

MR: I don't know . . . I'm not sure . . . but I could tell that they were scared when I couldn't breathe properly. You can tell when someone is scared. Not long after that I got even sicker; I had a high temperature and blinding headaches and I got terrible bruises from them constantly taking blood from me. My veins were wrecked, so they put a drip in my foot, and the only place they could get blood was from my femoral artery. I just lay there. I thought I was going to die.

The nurses were probably threatened by MR because she did not conceal her biological knowledge. She knew too much to be a 'good patient'. MR also had a way of exposing what the nurses did not know through her scientific questions, and this may have intimidated them. As MR said, she thought they were *'scared she might cark it'*. Everyone, it seemed, avoided asking questions and, because there were no answers, it was a time when the unspoken became the problematic, a time of silences.

BEING NOTHING: 'NO BODY'

MR's experience tells us she was reduced to nothing because sometimes she was not acknowledged as being there by the medical staff and everyone else was avoiding conversations with her. Imagine how it was for MR who had been on the ward for some months and she was becoming more and more disabled by the day. How frightening that must have been, lying in a bed without a diagnosis but feeling worse by the day. The hospital environment can lull people into a false sense of safety and security and I believe that this did happen to MR. This meant that her fear was somehow contained and she was able to be the patient believing that she would be helped. The doctors did not see MR very often during this time but her contact with the nurses increased as she needed more and more nursing care. The nurses began to refer to MR as 'basic nursing care' and this created yet another environment that made communication difficult for MR. In the next chapter MR tells us what it meant to her to be basic nursing care.

5

BEING 'BASIC NURSING CARE'

WHAT DID THE NURSES HAND OVER?

Waiting for a diagnosis became the time of silences when there were no answers to explain MR's deteriorating health. This was a difficult time for MR but it must also have become very difficult for the nurses, especially at the handover. How were the nurses to package and stereotype MR in the narrative of a handover? (Parker et al. 1992). Without a diagnosis what could they call her—full nursing care, a heavy patient or perhaps a quadriplegic of unknown origin? I guess all of these labels would have been used at some time by the nurses. Parker et al. (1992, p. 33) suggest that 'together, nurses at handover construct a collaborative narrative about the patients and like all narratives, this one has its heroes and its villains'. Before MR came to be known as a heavy patient, and perhaps a villain, she was referred to by the nurses as someone who was basic nursing care. As an expression this denigrates simultaneously the body and nursing (Lawler 1991, p. 31).

MR: I have often wanted to be a fly on the wall during a handover session. I would like to observe the dynamics, the conversations and the body language of the nurses. Handovers are supposed to be confidential but I often picked up on things that must have been said but, more importantly, on the things that were not said. I would have thought that things that had happened to me and how I felt would be passed on to the next nurse caring for me. When that didn't happen I would wonder what they did say about me and I always wondered why they did not ask me.

If you are in a hospital for more than a day at some stage the term handover will arise. Handovers are part of the culture of nursing and people who are outside of that culture never seem very sure of what and how information is gathered at these meetings. MR had been ill for some time so she knew that every day she would be discussed at least three times at a nursing handover. She learnt that what was said at the handover directly influenced some of the behaviour of the nurses towards her. She began to dread the passing on of information about her that she had no access to. While handover is presently being scrutinised by many scholars in terms of the effective use of time (Thurgood 1995; Prouse 1995; Matthews 1986; Monahan 1988) or as a cultural practice (Wiltshire and Parker 1996; McMahon 1993; Parker, Gardner and Wiltshire 1992; Parker and Gardner 1992) there is no mention in the literature as to how this cultural practice may affect a person's entire illness trajectory.

As I spend considerable time with students working through the language of handover and the subsequent labelling of people who are ill, I have come to realise that students come to view the handover as a rite of passage in nursing (McMahon 1994, p. 365). I believe that nurses need to meet, and that there should be spaces in hospitals where they can meet as do other health professionals. However, I am concerned that the nursing handover continues to be a strange mixture of nurses' stories and medical jargon that obscures the experiences of people who are ill and nurses themselves. MR wondered why the nurses never asked her how she might be feeling. She also raises the notion of confidentiality because in a small town sooner or later if you are discussed three times a day in an institution the information leaks into the community. Living within a close-knit community can be very supportive except when intimate details of your life are known by many people you have never even met. Confidentiality in a hospital is often a myth that most people, and especially nurses, perpetuate.

When the nurses referred to MR as basic nursing care in the handover they situated her discursively as being less important than some of the other people who were ill. This suggests that there is a hierarchy of care and MR as basic was therefore on the bottom. This language that some nurses use is far more denigrating and objectifying than medical discourse *because* it is part of the discourse of nursing. Even though Melia (in Lawler 1991, p. 31) states that 'basic nursing as a term has fallen into disrepute' it did not seem to be the case in relation to the nurses who cared for MR.

CARING FOR THE BODY

Previously I have proposed that we know very little about being a body (see also Nancy 1994). Nurses, however, engage in a highly complex, sophisticated activity that Lawler (1991) calls body care. Lawler (1991, p. 117) argues that for nurses 'to perform their work, therefore, they must overcome their own sociocultural backgrounds, and adjust to a particular professional subculture and its established methods that permits handling other people's bodies'. Furthermore Lawler (1991, p. 117) argues that nurses must 'confront the symbolism' attached to 'certain parts of the body' to perform body care. To reduce this highly contextualised sophisticated activity to the language of basic care is never to really understand or value how nurses manage people and their bodies.

I often hear colleagues refer to certain aspects of nursing care as basic. When nursing students first go into practice many registered nurses criticise them for not being able to do what they refer to as the basics. Nurses have not yet acknowledged their incredible expertise in handling people and their bodies. Students can learn a technical skill in a day but managing ill people requires experience over time. Exactly what do nurses mean when they say basic nursing care? It certainly implies far more than perhaps most nurses have ever imagined and is one of the metaphors in nursing that is problematic in the enculturation process of nursing students through rules and ritualised practices (Street 1992a, p. 9).

In subtle ways the expression of basic nursing care also reinforces the family symbolism within the hospital, the hierarchal structures of nursing that are dominated by medicine, the way gender influences values in the workplace and the Nightingale history of nursing. These issues highlight the way oppression operates in nursing and, once again, the way nurses participate willingly in their own domination. The socialisation of nurses into a culture of 'acceptance of taken-for-granted practices' (Perry 1986 in Street

1992a, p. 74) is exemplified every time I hear a nurse say basic, nursing, and care all in the same breath.

WATCHING AND LISTENING TO NURSES

So what did it mean to MR to be basic nursing care? She was unable to move her legs and had only minimal movement in her arms—her hands and her neck were very floppy. Since MR was confined to her bed or a chair because she could not move, the focus of her days became watching and listening to the nurses. From her position as basic nursing care she offers some insights into these experiences.

MR: Some nurses treated me as a person because I think some people just have an awareness of other people which translates in nursing to how they care for you. I have pictures in my head of the actions of many nurses, especially of nurses feeding people, and you think 'Why did they bother to become nurses?' I liked Jane, a new graduate, she was pretty impressive. When you are in a hospital room with three other people there's not much to look at, so everyone knows what's going on in the room and the way the nurse is interacting with all of the patients.

Benner and Wrubel (1989), and Lawler (1991) discuss how perhaps the experience of the nurse is crucial to how they might care for a person during illness. It is suggested that experienced nurses, referred to as 'experts' by Benner (1984), care for people in ways that are non-reductive which do not disembody the person (see Parker 1988; Parker 1991b; Gadow 1982; Colliere 1986; Wolf 1986; and Lawler 1991). Experienced nurses cared for MR but she considered very few of them as part of her embodiment. It was far more than the experience of the nurse that made them stand out for MR as experts.

The nurse who stood out for MR, a new graduate, was sensitively negotiating the very public space of a hospital ward. Through a process of enculturation many nurses, sadly, lose this sensitivity that MR noticed and appreciated. Using a Foucauldian analysis, Street (1992a) analyses some of the practices in nursing such as the full sponge to explain the process of enculturation. A full sponge, often referred to by nurses as hygiene, is thought to be the main component of basic nursing care. Street (1992a, p. 9) argues that the common sense knowledge that we would all have of how to wash our own bodies is 'transformed into a new ritual form through a requirement to unlearn common cultural practices and to re-learn the "hospital–ward way"' (Street 1992a, p. 9).

MR sometimes had the full sponge but often had a shower. This intimate time between her and a nurse was when she was to be at her most vulnerable. It is interesting then that registered nurses would often ask students or a newly graduated nurse to shower her. It was assumed that showering or washing MR was easy work and therefore manageable by someone new, because it was basic. Showering MR was a difficult and complex activity. It was when she was to be the most confronted by what she could no longer do for herself. MR remembers Jane again, the new graduate who had cared for her.

MR: Jane gave me great showers; she took the time and made sure that we weren't interrupted. Other nurses would poke their heads in and say that it was morning tea time or they would just interrupt to have a look at what was going on behind the door.

I too have been guilty of looking behind the screens or going into toilets or bathrooms when people have been exposed and vulnerable. As a clinical teacher I did this all of the time—a sort of overall surveillance of students and patients. I am always aware of the effect of my surveillance on the students' and the patients' behaviour. I have often been greeted with a person telling me that the student is doing a wonderful job, as a protective defensive response to my intrusion.

In particular though, what MR is referring to here, is that she was often showered during the designated morning tea period. Sometimes the nurses would relieve each other to take a tea break. This complex time of body care was when MR relied upon the nurse to be like extensions of her body. It is certainly an issue that nurses need to re-consider if they are going to listen to the concerns of people who are ill. It is a taken-for-granted yet inappropriate action for nurses to change over in the middle of what is a personal intimate time for any person. Jane knew how important this time was for MR from her everyday life, not from her experiences as a nurse and she would never leave MR until she was back in her bed or a chair. MR suggests that some people have this awareness of others which, if they are nurses, they translate into their practice.

MR has never forgotten Jane because she knew that for Jane not to go to tea at the designated time was to risk other nurses questioning her decision and sometimes they were aggressive towards her. The other issue that MR raises is how continuity of care is so important for her and people who are ill. When MR was tired and weak it was very stressful to have a different nurse every day and for her to have to explain how she wanted her body to be managed again and again. Jane would ask to care for MR so that they could continue their relationship therapeutically.

THE HABITS OF A LIFETIME

MR: Because I have been ill now for a long time I have to rely on the nurses. It has been essential that I change the habits of a lifetime. People who are chronically ill have to do this and it is a hard thing to accept. When I was first ill I thought that it was only temporary so handing over my body to be cared for was not as difficult as it is now. The transition to permanence is a time of turmoil at what is lost. I think it is basic to look after yourself. Certainly everyone does it to their own personal satisfaction and it is almost natural and automatic. You live with your own body and know it intimately well. People do develop their own routine of caring for themselves.

As a busy person I had evolved my own routine for washing, using my bowels, washing my hair, cleaning my teeth, dressing etc. This is all taken away from you when you lose your arms and legs. I think I became invisible to some nurses. I have also noticed that nurses will discuss other patients, sometimes in front of me. They forget that I'm in the room watching and listening. I have seen them not answer a call bell when it is rung depending on the patient who rings it. I decided to rarely use my bell, however, three and a half hours is the longest that I have had to wait for attention.

I remember a lady in a room with me was labelled as demanding. I wondered why the nurses did not tell this lady how busy they were rather than ignoring her. Hospital is filled with the unknown—you don't know what is happening to you. I think that people's demanding behaviour is a reflection of fear. I, myself, chose silence. I got treated the best if I were silent. If you take an interest in yourself in the hospital it seems to threaten the nurses.

While MR might argue that it is basic to look after oneself when they are well she indicates that all of this changed once she became ill. It is in this complex, contextual environment of illness that nurses must manage and assist people with what they have always done for themselves. As MR says, 'people are intimately connected to their bodies'. When a nurse takes over body care they must negotiate the fragile boundaries that exist between a person and their body because of an illness. What makes this even more difficult is that, as MR says, people are used to doing all of this automatically for themselves.

IN FOR INVESTIGATIONS

The days passed slowly for MR at this time and as her illness continued so did all of the diagnostic tests on her body. As the results came back, time and time again failing to reveal the cause of her illness, some nurses and other people avoided conversations with her. The nurses had said MR was 'in for investigation' but it was now becoming clear that the investigations were seemingly leading nowhere which is how they came to refer to her as 'basic nursing care'.

MR: I knew what many of the investigations that I had were for and, from listening and observing, I was able to follow what was transpiring. It got to the point where I was so desperate for a diagnosis that I would be disappointed when the tests were negative. Inconclusive results were something to be excited about. Being told nothing was more frustrating than having a diagnosis. Even if there was nothing specific to tell me they could have at least said something to reassure me. At least to express some concern or to tell me that they were not sure what was going on. It seemed that no one would talk to me about my illness.
    I was reminded of stories of doctors and relatives not telling someone that they had a terminal cancer or some other devastating disease to supposedly protect them. The thought did cross my mind that I had some horrible condition and they were waiting for me to die. I wonder if doctors ever stop to think of the mental anguish that a person goes through while they are waiting for a diagnosis. This continued with me for weeks then months then years. With a diagnosis comes certainty even if it does mean you are going to die. I think that the doctors were hoping that what was wrong with me was going to just go away of its own accord.

Even her regular flow of visitors slowed down and, as for many people who are chronically ill, she began to be an abandoned/neglected body.

MR: My social support became almost non-existent and yes sometimes I was very sad that people stopped coming to see me.

When I think back to this time I know that I did not visit MR as much as I would have liked and as she would have expected. I am not entirely sure why my visits slowed down, but I do remember how difficult it was to watch her slowly deteriorating. I think what I always avoided with MR was confronting the enormous issues that seemed to be developing around her as her illness progressed. Even when I did visit I would sometimes sit with her in silence. As she retreated into herself so, it would seem, did I. MR eventually stopped asking questions about her health and she was unusually silent. She stopped examining her results and charts and, at the same time, stopped telling me how she was feeling. She began to tell me of her confusion and of all of the things that were being done to her, rather than how she was feeling.

MR: I remember I was hypokalaemic at the time, that was one of the features. I was still having drips and vitalographs every day and peak flows, and my creatine phosphokinase levels went through the roof. There had been a flurry of tests because of my temperature and they put me on antibiotics, and I remember them saying 'You need these in case you get really sick with septicaemia'. I remember them saying that. I also remember the doctor asking me what I thought was wrong with me. I said, 'You're the doctor!' In the end I said to him, 'Well maybe I've got an atypical viral myopathy'.

The nurses didn't question any of it, and I kept telling them I couldn't swallow. I didn't know what was wrong with me. The breathing was a bother, but things were crowding in on me. I got angry because I was so weak I couldn't do much at all. I started to get angry with the way my doctor just came and stared at me from the end of the bed every day, without ever saying anything about what he thought. It was really weird. It was as if I wasn't there.

MR continued to objectify herself in relation to all of the tests she was having. She resented the doctor suddenly asking for her opinion on what might be wrong with her because she had never been asked for her opinion before. Until then she had been ignored, which explains her retort 'You're the doctor', although later she seized the opportunity (and control) to offer him a possible diagnosis. MR was placed in a difficult position to speak because of science and the doctor. Foucault has said 'Science . . . is literally a power that forces you to say certain things, if you are not to be disqualified not only as being wrong, but, more seriously than that, as being a charlatan' (Foucault in Minh-Ha 1991, p. 20). More importantly, science can be a power which intimidates and silences. The difficulty for MR was that she had no 'proof' to substantiate any diagnosis she might put forward.

MR also tells us that she was confused and angry with the doctor because all he did was stand at the end of the bed and look at her, without ever telling her what he saw or thought. This medical gaze to which Foucault (1975) refers to is the silence between the patient and the doctor, a clinical gaze, an observing gaze, that 'silently lets things surface without disturbing them with discourse' (Foucault 1975, p. xix). Through the silence, Foucault (1975, p. xix) argues that thoughts are synthesised into a medical discourse, and a discourse of disease emerges so the doctor can articulate 'what is seen and what is said'. But some doctors do not articulate what they see and, if they do, it may not often be to the person who is ill. MR describes being frustrated by the silence of the doctor and, although this gaze is argued by Foucault as non-reductive for the doctor, it is most certainly exclusionary for the patient.

NOT ALL STORIES ARE 'GOOD'

Many of the stories that MR tells when she recalls this time of silence are stories that nurses may find unsettling to read. At first I found it difficult to write these experiences down. The history of nursing and women has made it difficult at times for nurses to feel positive about nursing. As a result of this many nurses have only recently begun to recognise and value the contribution they make to health care. Nursing scholars have appropriately concentrated on the stories that help nurses to develop a confidence in themselves and nursing. Therefore nurses are not often confronted with a story such as MR's that requires an acknowledgment that perhaps many aspects of nursing need to be scrutinised, understood and changed.

Being 'Basic Nursing Care'

When people try to voice their negative experiences of receiving health care services it is usually in the form of a complaint to management. Nurses have learned that, if there are complaints from 'patients' or their relatives, they may be victimised and blamed inappropriately. For example when someone complains about the nursing care often the response of the nurses is to become even more ritualised and routine with their practices. As a result nurses may lose their remarkable creativity that only comes about when they are confident to blur the institutional boundaries that constrain their practice. For protection nurses wrap themselves in a cocoon of protocols and rituals where people and their bodies are lost and silenced.

It is apparent, on some wards, that at some time a nurse has been blamed or victimised because there are some unusual policies in place. For example nurses will not be giving out certain medications because of an historical drug error or they will not be making decisions on wound care. In fact they may not be making many autonomous decisions at all. In comparison if doctors restricted their clinical practices because of these types of incidents little would be going on in hospitals.

The problem is that nurses are not in the habit of evaluating their practice through the patients' experiences or peer review. Nurses are often unaware of how a person has experienced nursing care while they were in hospital. Of course, some people will and do express to nurses how they feel about the interactions they have with them. It may be in a look or a touch or they talk to the nurse about the difference they have made to their illness experience.

MR: During the past years I have observed hundreds of nurses going about their work. They are a fascinating breed and there are many different ways in which they interact with the patient. I could not say that I have been impressed with much of the treatment or care I have seen nurses involved in. This doesn't just apply to myself, but to many of my fellow patients. I guess there is always a certain camaraderie between patients and you feel protective towards each other. Some treatment could only be described as distressing to observe.

I remember there was a person on the ward who had failed in a suicide attempt and had done themselves a great deal of damage. The way that the nurses spoke about this person made me so angry. Some refused to look after the patient and most spoke with judgmental overtones. That person must have felt similar vibes to me.

JUST A HEAD

Because I had been around on the ward for a while I got the impression that the nurses were fed up with looking after me. I was on a cancer (oncology) ward and some nurses actually told me that they only liked looking after cancer patients. My so-called primary nurse was one of them. It was hardly my fault that I spent some time on the oncology ward; the patient doesn't get to choose. In my experience, the 'ideal' patient is one who is self-caring, only requires medication and is compliant by remaining quiet. A patient, such as myself, who requires help with basically everything is not desirable.

I don't think the caring aspect of nursing is learned from experiences of nursing but is an innate part of the nurse's personality.

MR believes that the ability to care is innate. While I understand what she means, suggestions such as this can create a dilemma similar to that created when people imply that some women are 'born nurses' (see Street 1992b, p. 183). One of the consequences of such a statement is the implication that anyone with a little common sense can become a nurse.

In a similar vein Taylor (1994) theorises how problematic the taken-for-granted knowledges are in nursing when she analyses what she refers to as the ordinariness in nursing in her doctoral study. Taylor (1994, p. 230) tells us: 'When things appear familiar and apparently common place we may tend to take them for granted, and discount them as being relatively unimportant. The simple things can be among the most instructive agents in gaining wisdom and experience. I contend that ordinariness is one such case.'

The longer that MR was in hospital the more the nurses took for granted her weak and flaccid body. Likewise MR had stopped asking questions and she found that her experiences as a patient were more positive if she was silent. She got used to things such as not being able to communicate with the outside world because there was not a phone that she could use. There was one period when the nurses told me that the phone was broken and she did not talk with anyone on the phone for three months. Initially MR and others complained but it soon became a taken-for-granted that there was no phone on the ward for patients.

WHAT DID THE DOCTORS SEE?

Oliver Sacks, Tony Moore and Arthur Frank all experienced the same silence and loss of voice that MR talks about. MR says that she was treated as if she was not there and that the doctors and the nurses avoided having conversations with her. With no medical diagnosis the doctors silently observed her from the end of the bed and the nurses were also silenced because they were unable to express what they saw and heard. So, if medical discourse incorporates 'a perpetual and objectively based correlation of the visible and the expressible' as Foucault (1975, p. 196) suggests, what did the doctors see, and what did they say about what they saw? The visible signs of a body losing tone and function were there, doctors could see the clinical changes on the surface of MR's body. Even if the diagnostic test results were abnormal they could now be explained as a result of MR's immobility. There was no pathology to give language to MR's illness and legitimacy to her being a patient.

As such the abyss beneath her illness, that is the illness itself, had no name and could not be revealed through language. Doctors had said nothing to MR because they had nothing to say. The syntactical organisation of disease into language, that would render MR an object of science through a discursive existence, could not occur. At this point it would seem that MR was caught between the space of being enfleshed or disembodied, or as Laqueur (1990, p. 12) puts it, between 'an extraordinary, fragile, feeling, transient mass of flesh that we are familiar with and the cultural meanings that we as bodies are so bound to'. Part of the cultural meanings that bodies are bound to is the relationship between food and the body. In the next chapter I discuss how MR struggled with this relationship in relation to the cultural connections between eating, food and the body.

6

BEING UNABLE TO EAT

THE SYMBOLISM OF FOOD

In reading this chapter on being unable to eat it is important to recall that MR has a background in the science of nutrition. This shapes her experiences and reflections when she is remembering issues of herself and food. The work of Deborah Lupton is used in this chapter because she makes the important distinction between a nutritionist's interests in diet and the conceptual differences between their concerns and those of anthropologists and sociologists (Lupton 1996, p. 7). Nurses rarely work with the interests of anthropologists and sociologists rather, they tend to have a 'scientific' approach in regard to ill people and food (White 1991). That is, food is seen as fuel for the biological body, and the symbolic nature of food is not usually considered.

This approach is argued by Lupton (1996, p. 7) to be highly problematic because 'food practices' are 'far more complex than a simple nutritional or biological perspective would allow'. Before MR became ill she had wanted to lose weight and get fit in order to look a particular way. The self-regulating practices of dieting and exercising and the quest for the 'thin ideal' are the hallmark traits of contemporary femininity. Individual approaches to dieting and exercise, however, can be different. A diet, to MR, was about assessing the body and energy expenditure, eating healthy food and exercising to lose and then maintain an ideal weight. When MR and I were dieting she measured and weighed me in order to work out a plan for me to follow to lose weight. Since I considered her to be the expert on food this approach suited me because I could hand my body over to MR and I did not have to determine the rules to discipline my body, just follow them.

If I diet by myself I seem to enter into a battle with my body which is extremely destructive in my day to day living. For example, I find it difficult to buy food or cook because I develop a fear that I will lose control and buy and eat fattening food. MR, on the other hand, talked more about food and cooking and all the great food we could eat when we decided to go on a diet together. She did not see diet as deprivation, as I did, rather as alteration of a lifestyle. When we were exercising MR began to cook some really interesting food and brought it in to work for us. Her internalised scientific belief that food was not the enemy was based upon the belief that you need to understand how the nutrients released from food 'interact with the physiological characteristics of the eater' (Khare 1980 in Lupton 1996, p. 7). By controlling the type of food that is eaten it is thought that one can control the self. Nutritionists tend to believe that we all need scientific knowledge about the nutritional value of food to make informed healthy choices on what to eat.

FAMILY, FOOD AND GENDER

Food habits and practices are behaviours that have been internalised throughout life and this conscious moulding of our bodies, that Foucault (1988) would call 'technologies of the self', accounts for the ways that people construct and express subjectivity. When MR became ill there was a disruption in her ability to maintain her subjectivity when food and eating practices were no longer incorporated into her experiences of living. In hospital what she ate and how much she was offered were limited by the hospital menu. As her illness progressed MR eventually lost her ability to swallow and therefore to eat. Here MR begins to discuss her relationship with food after she became ill.

MR: Eating and my nutritional status have remained a constant problem throughout my illness. Prior to my illness I had always managed to eat very well. However, when you feel like shit you don't really feel all that much like eating but I had always managed to eat very well prior to my illness. Since I have been ill I have been starved and forced to eat. For example, at one stage they said to me 'If you don't eat, you will have to leave'. I would have to say that the years of healthy eating were to hold me in good stead for the months, then the years of deprivation of adequate nutrition. In fact it probably saved my life. However, my relationship with food and attitude towards eating has been irrevocably damaged as a result of seemingly relentless assaults or deprivations involving food, eating and provision of adequate nutrition.

MR tells us that her nutritional status has been a problem for a variety of reasons. She has been unable to eat sometimes because she has been too ill and then she has become worried about her health and wellbeing to the extent that she believed that her body was damaged because of inadequate nutrition. She argues that she was forced to eat. This does not mean that someone forced food into her but rather that she was coerced into eating. MR believed that eating all of the food she was given ensured that she was still going to be cared for in a particular way. If MR did not eat all of the food provided she was not seen to be doing her part in helping herself 'get better'. In many families children are coerced by parents to eat all of their meals. In much the same way, if MR was seen to be eating her meals she implies that it influenced the nurses and how they would care for her. Parents reward and punish children in much the same way concerning food.

The sociology of food in acute hospital settings is discussed by Fran McInerney (1992). The analysis that McInerney (1992, p. 1271) engages in relates to people living with cancer. Her analysis explores the sociology of food, the role of gender and the acute hospital and she argues that in the hospital there is a cultural replication of the family (McInerney 1992, p. 1275). It is the powerful symbols of family, food and gender that become problematic for MR while she is in hospital. Within the family, women who are wives and mothers are central to preparing food and feeding the family. Being a 'good' wife or 'good' mother is often equated with how well a women can cook or her interest in what all of the family eats. Being a 'good nurse' can be equated to the nurse whose patient eats all of their food.

According to Lupton (1996, pp. 52, 53) the mother usually exerts domination over the eating habits of children in families.

The 'clean your plate or else' syndrome is a memory many people share from childhood (Lupton 1996, p. 52). Food and eating are incorporated into childhood memories often in the context of the family. Therefore these memories are bound with emotion for all of us. I remember meal times in my own family where the expectation was that we had to eat everything on our plates. Rejecting a meal was also to reject my mother's cooking and my parents' wisdom on what I needed to consume to become a healthy adult. As an adult I still remember some family meal times with negative emotions.

The differential power relations between parents and children is analogous to nurses and patients. Game and Pringle (1983) refer to this analogy in their work and Garmanikow (1978) refers to the gender relations in families that are replicated within the hospital setting by nurses and doctors. MR equated concern by nurses and doctors over her nutritional status with being cared for. Some nurses struggled with MR's weight loss and treated her as the naughty child who would not eat up her dinner. I heard a nurse say to her one day *'You're going to be a good girl for me, aren't you, and eat up all of your dinner'*. Saying this in front of me, the visitor, ensured that I also pressured MR to eat and I stayed with her while she ate every mouthful.

In my early days of nursing I remember watching a close friend and nurse, Sue, feed an elderly woman until she gagged and spat food all over her. The woman had suffered a stroke and was crying as she was being fed. Sue was angry with the woman and she told her she would 'never get better if she did not eat up'. Sue believed that she was doing the 'right thing' as a nurse and later did the same to her children as a mother. After all she had probably been treated in much the same way by her parents who had probably believed that it was for 'her own good'.

BEING A 'FEED'

Meal times in hospitals conjure up all sorts of memories for me as a nurse. I remember the times when I had to dish up the meals in an aged care setting. The smell of the food and the look of it remain my most unpleasant memories of food. Elderly people filled the room in armchairs with fixed tables. They had on large bibs and it was my job to serve up dinner and then, somehow, simultaneously to feed about ten people. I would move from person to person giving one spoonful at a time. I remember that the nurses would refer to people at the handover as 'feeds'. Being a feed is often a component of being basic care and eventually MR came to be known as both.

MR: From the time I was in ICU my problems with food began because for the first three weeks of my illness I did not receive any form of nutrition. Needless to say I started to lose a substantial amount of weight. My problems with food were exacerbated by the gradual loss of my ability to swallow, as the effects of my illness became widespread throughout my increasingly alien body. I had trouble with swallowing any of my tablets and seemed to have difficulty swallowing my saliva. They investigated all of these problems. I had fluoroscopy studies in which you are required to take mouthfuls of barium of differing consistencies and you are X-ray filmed swallowing them. I saw the Ear Nose and Throat specialist who was unable to find any obvious defects in the structure of my larynx, so it was suggested the problem was of neurological origin.

I had intravenous fluids but I became obsessed with eating. I started to have hallucinations about food which were so real that every sensation about food was aroused. I hallucinated about a meat pie of all things—it is still really clear in my mind. The colours were vivid—golden brown and rich red. It smelled hot and fresh. There was one bite out of it and the sauce and meat were spilling down my hand. It is ironic that I don't even like meat pies.

The smell of a meat pie evoked memories for MR that were pleasant. Lupton (1996, p. 32) proposes that 'there is a strong relationship between memory and the emotional dimensions of food'. MR loves football so perhaps the smell of a meat pie transports her back to Saturdays at the football, when she was well and happy, and the smell of meat pies pervaded the air. I can certainly be reminded of pleasant times via the smell of meat pies although I do not like them. Perhaps my dislike of meat pies, though, is because I see them as bad food. For me, eating a meat pie, especially in public, is symbolic of moral weakness. Meat, according to Lupton (1996, p. 29), has many connotations attached to it that incorporate aspects of 'goodness' and 'badness'. A meat pie, however, is also a fast food and therefore seen by many people as unhealthy food that is not good for you.

Not long after MR dreamt of the meat pie she had an encounter with some jelly. Although jelly is an ideal food for those having difficulty swallowing it also has a very sweet, lolly-like smell which reminds many people of their childhood. I associate jelly with my mother caring for me, because I had it when I was ill or for special occasions when my mother would add fruit to it. From her childhood MR remembers jelly ponds with chocolate frogs in it and games with wibbly wobbly jelly. The smell of jelly evoked some strong emotional memories for MR.

MR: I did have the nasogastric tube and enteral feeding for a while and then I had swallowing lessons with the speech pathologist. One day they brought in some raspberry jelly. I stared at the bowls of jelly and breathed in the raspberry fumes. I was salivating and I could almost taste it. After a while the nurses removed the jelly because they said that the doctors had said that the risk of aspiration was too great.

Eventually I lost my appetite and found that I could go for days without eating.

Turner (1992, p. 226) in his discussion of anorexia argues that 'loss of appetite is phenomenologically parallel to loss of speech, and both conditions point to the absence of social voice'. While Turner is considering anorexic behaviour in people who have eating disorders his analysis can be meaningful in relation to MR's experiences. She was to lose both her appetite and her ability to voice her opinions. MacSween (1995, p. 94), in her analysis of anorexia, argues that in anorexia there is an 'absolute opposition between appetite and "self"'. She links appetite with the desiring body as opposed to the body that wants and needs nothing. MR tells us that she lost her appetite and found, as people with anorexia do, that she could go for days without eating.

MR: Later I was to regain some of my ability to swallow and I could eat a small amount of vitamised food. The dietitian gave up on me though and I would see her going past my door and she would look at me with an air of disgust. My friends tried to talk with and see the dietitian and the doctors but they were told it was none of their concern. As a patient I couldn't speak for myself any more and no one could on my behalf.

MR thought that the dietitian had given up because she had stopped seeing her. She thought that she was angry with her for not eating and swallowing and the punishment was to be no more treatment.

MR: The dietitian told me that the nurses had told her I had refused a nasogastric tube. I don't remember doing that but maybe that's why she was angry with me.

SKIN AND BONE

As time passed MR's body began to look ravaged from her illness, immobility and lack of nutrition. She began to get angry and frustrated with the way that she looked.

MR: I not only felt like shit I looked like shit. I was just skin and bone. My Ethiopian look I called it. All of those years of work to produce a well muscled, athletic body were destroyed in a few short weeks. I found my profoundly wasted legs distressing. I still detest looking at my limbs protruding from the end of my torso. I avoid mirrors whenever possible. I worried that I would die from starvation. No-one ever seemed concerned about my nutrition. If you cannot feed yourself then, in a hospital, you get three chances a day to eat and the nurses got sick of how slow I was eating. I would often say I was full to get the nurses away from me. Friends came in to feed me.

The sense of alienation and separation from her body that MR began to experience from not eating is argued, by Lupton (1996, p. 141), to be a phenomenon also experienced by people with eating disorders. Not being able to eat contributed to the disembodiment that MR experienced.

MR: I continued with the speech pathologist and the occupational therapist who made me a special hand strap for my spoon. I could drag mush from the plate on to my chest and then to my mouth. I lost most of it on the way but I was determined to do this for myself. Sometimes I would have a spasm and the food flew off the spoon.

There were times that I would feel sick just looking at the pulverised blobs of food that MR was offered. Since she was in a room with three other people, who all struggled to eat their meals, it was not conducive to enjoying food. Making vitamised food look appetising is difficult and the plastic tray and bowls did not help. The food would often go cold because there were not enough nurses to feed everyone. The aroma of the food would mix with the smell of people, illness and hospitals—which did not help to stimulate appetites. MR regarded meal times as a time to persist at feeding herself rather than to enjoy her food. Thus MR remembers meal times as a time when she would try to regain her ability to feed herself again.

MR: When I went to rehabilitation, there was a sudden flurry of interest again in my body weight and nutritional status. I was weighed—I had lost thirty kilos at one time in nine weeks. Eventually they decided to assist my eating by strapping me upright in a chair. To do this they used velcro around my head. I looked like an anorexic Jane Fonda with a headband. This might sound fine in theory but this was one of the worse experiences of my life. It was total humiliation. I sat in the middle of the ward and everyone could see me. The first time I sat there silently crying and on display for all to see. Once I was left there for hours because they forgot me. I hated my friends seeing me like that in the pink torture chair.

For the first time MR likens her body to that of someone with anorexia. Interestingly it is Jane Fonda that she refers to—Jane Fonda has became a popular symbol of slenderness attained through diet and exercise regimes through her videos. The images of Fonda working out strapped to gym equipment are for MR, superimposed with the images of anorexia. MR recognises the fragile boundaries that exist between the thin but fit body moulded through diet and exercise and the disciplinary practices of starving the body. Bordo (1989, p. 18) would argue that 'food is not the real issue here', rather the issue of control of the female appetite. Bordo (1989, pp. 22–3) further argues that anorexia can begin 'as a fairly moderate diet regime'. MR had lost her appetite and her desire to eat and this became etched upon her body. She was aware that she now embodied an anorexic look but she would have preferred the Jane Fonda look.

MR remembers her weight loss and the fact that the doctors and nurses were interested in how much she weighed. While she was pleased that they were taking an interest in her body again she was very unhappy to be strapped into a chair for eating. The chair came to represent many things to MR. Strapped around the head she looked as if she was ready for execution and, as she says, she hated being on display in the middle of the room. MR did not want to be a captive in the chair when her friends came to visit. It made the interactions with friends strained because she was self-conscious about her body and how she looked. When MR wrote the story of the pink torture chair it stood out for me because she said that she cried in the chair and that she cried alone and silently.

NOT A MERRY CHRISTMAS

MR: My first Christmas in hospital was not merry for me. I had not celebrated Christmas for some years because I considered it to be too commercial and burdensome. I certainly did not want it imposed upon me. I was expected to gather with five other patients in the dining room with all of the trimmings. Out came the pink chair and the nurses carried me to the table in it. Pureed Christmas lunch just did not seem the same. There were two pale coloured blobs, possibly turkey and potato, one green blob and two orange blobs. I had only a couple of mouthfuls before I choked. I just couldn't bring myself to eat any more after that. The nurses seemed to be enjoying the lunch and I was made to sit through a replay of *Carols by Candlelight*. Hell, even if it exists, could not compare to this Christmas.

Christmas dinners, according to Lupton (1996, p. 63), 'serve a similar function to an archetypal "family meal"'. She proposes at the heart of this domestic ritual that there is 'the relationship of parents with children'. Is it any wonder then that being ill in a hospital at Christmas will conjure up strong emotions. Nurses do try to reproduce the feeling of festivity and family but they can go home to their families for the 'real' celebration after work.

The tension and painful remembering that MR experienced at Christmas may not have been realised by the nurses. I have worked many shifts at Christmas and was encouraged to put on Christmas socks, or maybe a badge or Christmas earrings. I did not really appreciate the pain that Christmas can bring to people trapped in institutions because I was desperately trying to keep the mythology of Christmas alive. The emotional experiences that are seemingly hidden all year intensify at Christmas and that emotion can be experienced as physical pain. MR experienced much the same and being made to sit at the table with everyone was deeply distressing for her.

Meal times for MR were, as for everyone, probably always charged with different emotions. Here she remembers the meal times she enjoyed.

MR: There was one very social occasion that I did enjoy. Sometimes a friend and I would get the nurse to order a family-sized pizza with extra hot chilli. It was so hot we could barely eat but it was a challenge to eat some of it on our own. It was a great competition which usually ended with hysterical laughter and pizza on the floor.

On these occasions MR could exercise some control. She could ask the nurse to order the food and at the same time it would seem that to order a pizza with hot chilli when she was on a pureed diet was possibly an enjoyable act of defiance. MR indicates that the staff thought that she was deliberately not eating because of the many stories that she makes reference to such as the following.

MR: Once the director of the unit came to see me and she said that I would have to leave if I did not start eating properly. When the next large meal came in I gave part of it to my friend to take home for her cat. I also hid food whenever I could and they never twigged. I was weighed bi-weekly.

FOOD IN A BAG

Hiding food is behaviour that is often discussed in relation to people who are living with anorexia and was most certainly an issue of control and autonomy for MR. Many women with anorexia, interviewed by MacSween (1995), discuss their feelings of powerlessness and the need to exert some control. In hiding her food MR achieved a sense of power over those seeking to control her body. When she was artificially fed, this battle between the nurses and MR, stopped. The bags of fluid (food) were administered by the nurses as if they were medications. Thus the symbolism of food was removed from her sense of self and the issue of when and how much she ate was not an issue.

MR: I was able to go home at one stage when I was being artificially fed. For this to happen the community nurses had to be organised to maintain the feeds because the carers were not permitted to handle them. Being artificially fed enabled my poor nutritional status to recover but then I got an infection in my stoma. I ended up back in hospital to get a more appropriate feeding-tube. Sometimes the tube would block and disconnect, pumping feed into my bed whilst my gut contents would pour out the tube. If I were asleep I would not know this was happening. My poor depleted body—it was relentless, never ending. I felt dreadfully ill and could see no end to my situation until, maybe, I died some horrible death. I was terrified that I was going to end up being kept alive by a machine with no escape.

MR talks about her poor depleted body as if it was separate to herself. I visited her one day after her tube had become disconnected and she was really distressed because she had been asleep when her gastric contents had emptied into her bed. She had to lie in the wet bed until the nurse came on her rounds as she could not reconnect it herself. Being ill at home presented MR with a multitude of challenges but she persevered because she much preferred to be in her own home. Sometimes, however, she became too ill to manage.

MR: Once I got very sick on one of the times I tried to be at home. Denise took me back into the hospital. They seemed to take notice of me this time and great concern was shown for my weight loss and so I had enteral feeds again for a couple of months. Then all the problems started again and they removed the tube and sent me back to rehab to be fed by the nurses again. This was never successful and I remember a nurse telling me I was being silly when I did not swallow properly. She would refuse to feed me and would walk off.

As soon as MR was being fed again by the nurses the interactions that mimic parents and children resumed. For this reason, and because of her concern that she was not receiving adequate nutrition, she preferred to be artificially fed. Then the nurses were somewhat removed from her nutrition in that they administered the feeds in the same way as medications prescribed by doctors. This also ensured that there were fewer interactions between the nursing staff and MR, as they did not have to feed her.

The connections between food, subjectivity and embodiment are very complex but an area that needs to be considered especially by nurses. Unfortunately because nutrition is seen as a science, cultural practices and meanings around food are not seen as part of a person's embodiment. MR is a person who loves food and entertaining, and she is a wonderful cook. Since MR has been ill she has gradually lost her cultural connections to food—yet another loss in her life.

Being unable to eat

Throughout all of the experiences that MR had as her body changed the struggle to find out why she was so ill continued—her quest for a diagnosis continued. As you will read in the next chapter, without a diagnosis MR began to experience being disembodied, describing herself as just a head.

7

BEING 'JUST A HEAD'

NURSES AS ARMS AND LEGS

Days had become weeks and weeks had become months, summer had come and MR was no better, she was still deteriorating. Often alone now MR would contemplate how her world had changed. As she became weaker she gradually began to disengage from her body but she was philosophical about what was happening to her.

MR: I don't know what I believe any more about the mind and the body. Sometimes I am really surprised by my body. It's hard to explain, but I sort of think 'Oh, it's me. Is that part of me?' It's very strange; so I guess, for me, my mind is separate to my body. I feel very detached and I didn't feel like this when I was well. Sometimes I was made to feel as if I wasn't a person.

I really get nurses and carers to look after my body well. I get oil rubbed into my skin. I ask to be exercised. I make sure they use sterile techniques with catheters and that they do every thing properly—that they wash me properly. I have evolved how we do things. I hate it when I have new people because I have to train them. The carers and nurses are like my arms and legs; the ones I have had for a while just do everything automatically—they do all these things, so we can talk about other things.

It was this conversation that first enabled MR and me to begin to talk about what her illness actually meant to her. When she had first described herself as just a head I had asked her questions about nurses and how they cared for her. Initially I was unsure of how to respond, but since then we have continued to use the explicit Cartesian language that MR uses to explore what being just a head might mean to her. Most people respond to MR by saying that she is more than just a head and it has probably been the nurses who have been most confronted by her remarks. I think that this is probably because they come to know MR as a person and it is therefore difficult for them to reduce what they see, touch and experience every day as MR to a head.

RE-EMBODIED AS A HEAD

MR's story so far has been one of her desperately seeking an identity through a medical diagnosis. She had given over her body for investigation and to some extent had investigated her own body in the hope she would find answers to explain her illness. As time passed and neither she nor the doctors found any explanations she became silent and disembodied. As MR lost her feeling for her body she indicates that she became re-embodied as just a head. She argues that as she lost her body her illness forced her to make the split between mind and body in becoming just a head. However, as just a head she was able to conceive the nurses as extensions of her 'self' so she could be more than just the head. She describes the nurses as part of her body when she says that they were 'like my arms and legs'. In this sense she was re-embodied.

By constructing herself as a head, MR constructs the body as the 'negative other of mind' (Cranny-Francis 1995, p. 3). According to Cranny-Francis (1995, p. 3) 'the consequences of this negative valorisation of body are far reaching'. MR dismisses bodily activity to become just a head. As a result of this dualism MR is limited or confined by her body, and her body can be thought of as trapping or imprisoning her mind (Cranny-Francis 1995, p. 4). It is the process of the objectification of MR's body which eventually renders her as 'no body' that is so confronting. MR has made explicit the mind–body dualism through her illness experience.

MR: It has been through my illness that I became, and still see myself as, just a head. I do acknowledge that I have a body, but I don't feel that it is part of me. Rather it is like something material that I own, like a house or a car. To be frank, my regard for my body isn't something personal any more. Maybe this is how I protect myself because I can't stand the thought of what my body has become.

My body has been extensively studied and investigated and invaded periodically throughout my illness. Interest waxed and waned in the search for a definitive diagnosis. I have certainly stood apart from my body to examine and analyse it. In my own research with people I enjoyed the contact and individuality of my subjects. However I recognise that ultimately I reduced them to numbers, categories and statistics. In much the same way I have now become a patient with a number and results that are compared to other results and numbers but not to other people.

I think that the person has been forgotten by medical science and, in my case I am a person who has forgotten their body. I guess that my body was forgotten by medicine because I did not fit into one of the neat medical pigeonholes. There were so many pieces to the puzzle of me but no permutation or combination could form a recognisable picture. Thus my body in pieces was cast into the shunned wilderness world of the psychosomatic. The machine of medicine could never admit they just didn't know.

I said that the nurses were like extensions of my arms and legs and that was because they had to meet all of my bodily needs. On the occasions that I did get home the carers were able to be my arms and legs more easily. This was probably because there were less of them for me to conceive as extensions. I had many nurses care for me over time and so it is difficult to even remember them all. I could somehow direct the carers more whereas the nurses had long since decided how something should be done. I mean they have decided how to wash you or wipe your bottom before you get the chance to tell them. A few might listen to me but surely I am in the best position to know what should be done for me and how it should be done. Some nurses didn't take my suggestions kindly and did it their way regardless.

I have resorted to joking with the nurses and saying that my buttocks are tattooed with 'wipe' on one cheek and 'properly' on the other. I always thought that you would care for others how you might yourself or your own family. However, I cannot afford to alienate the nurses and so I compromise—that's all I can do. Experience and observation has taught me that demanding patients get less done for them than the compliant or passive patient. About the only thing I have always insisted on is that the nurses turn me every two or three hours to prevent pressure sores. I forget these days to even ask for some of the many little things to be done that you would automatically do for yourself. I don't remember to ask a nurse to brush my teeth if they forget to. I usually remember in the middle of the night that my teeth are dirty. Luckily I've got friends who are nurses who have always done some of these things for me.

THE 'DOCILE' VISITOR

Although it can be difficult for nurses to negotiate the extent of the nursing care that they will give, clearly it is essential to keep negotiating nursing care with the person being cared for and family and friends. Nurses are mindful that a different network of people will care for a person in the community once they leave the hospital. MR was always talking about going home and so she let some friends assist her with some of the intimate details of her body care. In the same way that ill people handover their bodies to be cared for by nurses, nurses hand them back when the time is right or, depending on the person, they may hand some of the body care over to relatives and friends. It is incredibly complex to get this balance right to suit all of the people involved. I was never one of the friends that got involved in the body care of MR. I had already discovered that whenever I asked questions about MR that there were consequences and this had scared me off doing anything for her. I am amazed when I look back at my behaviour.

One incident that affected me occurred one evening when I visited MR. The nurses were having a particularly bad evening and there was not enough of them to care for all of the patients. MR's catheter bag was about to explode and I went to tell a nurse, because if I emptied it myself they might accuse me of interfering. When I found the nurse she said to me 'MR? *Who is she?*' I pointed to her bed and she rolled her eyes and became very angry telling me how busy they were. I felt confronted and found myself saying that I recognised they were busy and that I could empty the bag—but perhaps it was inappropriate to yell at me; and I walked away. The nurse yelled after me, 'And *you are . . . ?*' I turned and said *'Denise Fassett'*. She stared at me in disbelief as it registered that I was not only also a nurse but a suspect university lecturer (from 'out there'). The next day the nurses had written down the occasion as an incident that somehow 'blamed' me (just in case I should complain) and sent it to the director of the area. I can only assume that they were feeling guilty to document at some length why they had not been able to empty a catheter bag. This and many other experiences, including being with MR when she first became ill, silenced the interactions that I was prepared to have with anyone, including MR, in the hospital.

THE ONLY 'PRIVATE THING' LEFT

MR: I now believe that surely no illness is purely of mind or body—there are elements of both in all illnesses. What is medicine so afraid of? Why is it so afraid of people like me? How can anyone argue that what happens to the body will not affect the mind or vice versa? What would you expect if one day you were well and then you were very ill? Am I not to be affected by this? Now, some years later, do you expect that I would be unaffected by the treatment that has been dealt out to me in institutional settings? Some of the treatment towards me has been outrageous.

I am a private person but can no longer act so now that I am ill. My illness has confronted both my independence and my privacy. It hardly bothers me now who sees my body because I simply have no choice. Illness is a bewildering and an isolating state and people are depersonalised. Some people expose their souls to nurses but I don't think that I ever have. My father tends to tell my story or his story of me to the nurses. He bails up the nurses in the corridor and talks to them. I am too worried about being discussed to reveal too much too them.

I have been sick for a long time so, in the end, I have lost my privacy and with it my dignity. I'm not sure whether comfortable is the right word for how I feel about being seen naked or having nurses touch and wash me. I just switch off—one of the advantages of being just a head.

Gatens (1996, p. 35) argues that 'we may think of our own bodies as the most private of all our "possessions", but in fact the body has about it an eerie anonymity and otherness that is especially felt at times of illness'. In a sense then Gatens is suggesting a similar concept to that of MR when she says she could no longer reclaim her body back because it was not part of her. Illness, according to Gatens (1996, p. 35), may be a time when 'we feel alienated from our social surroundings and times at which we are vulnerable to objectification by others'.

MR says that illness is isolating and depersonalising and suggests that the alienation that she experiences from her body is similar to the alienation that she experiences from society. Being part of society as a person with a chronic illness is extremely difficult, but to be chronically ill without a diagnosis is to be also alienated from the objectification of the body that dominates the way people experience illness. Much of the critique of the objectification of people and their bodies highlights the incompatibility of medicine and the illness experience. MR has discussed being the body object, the body of science, but, paradoxically, without a diagnosis MR is alienated from a certain objectivity that might have enabled her to make sense of her illness experience.

AN IN-BETWEEN SPACE

I have difficulty in explaining the way that MR describes her embodiment. Parker (1997, p. 25) refers to the way Merleau-Ponty describes embodiment 'as an interfolding of being and world'. She argues that 'this understanding of the body breaks down the Cartesian binary division between body and mind'. In trying to theorise how MR tells us that she is embodied as a head it seems that she is speaking from a space of resistance, an in-between space. It is an in-between space because 'a number of temporalities intersect' (Parker 1997, p. 22). MR has come to inhabit this space through her experiences of alienation from her body and society. By describing herself as just a head she forces us to consider and confront the binary divisions between body and mind. Thus by using the Cartesian language that in itself constitutes a fragmented body she challenges us all to consider the way the body is conceived by society.

Drawing on the work of Minh-Ha (1992), Parker (1997, p. 22) discusses how she believes that nurses also assume a position of in-between since they speak the 'voices of medicine, nursing, institution and patient'. In this sense she argues that nurses are hybrid. Parker (1997, p. 22) is making the point that rather than a nurse being 'confused and disorientated by this multivocality' they can 'assume a position in-between' to come to new understandings with that which has previously been hidden.

Lawler (1997, p. 37) argues that 'scientific discourse does not allow the person to enter the story, except in the passive voice and, consequently, it does not allow for embodiment or the non material world'. I believe that, initially, much of MR's story of her illness shaped her experiences of embodiment as she desperately tried to enter the medical story. Her only voice was passive but, eventually with no diagnosis, her passive voice was silenced. In this text MR enters the story through language that forces people to confront her embodiment as just a head and more importantly they are forced to think about MR the person.

REFLECTING THE BODY

MR: I have grieved so long and so hard for all of my losses and for the loss of not being able to care for myself. Becoming a head has made this easier. This doesn't mean that I don't care what happens to my body. If my body is not cared for then it threatens the health of my head. My head, or I guess my mind, is the only thing that I have left. It is difficult to maintain some pride in how I look now. I never look in a mirror any more because I know I won't like what I see. To be honest, I've never been that happy with the way that I look.

MR made another interesting comment about looking into a mirror. She said that when I went to visit her she would study my face to try to read what my reactions were to her body. It would seem that MR thought that I acted as a mirror because she said that she could see her body reflected in my face. I have not become accustomed to seeing MR as she is now. Knowing a person's history enables one to see more than the actual moment before you. Sometimes, on looking at MR I could visualise her walking with me or teaching at work. There was the time when she had broken her leg and was in plaster and I had asked her to take a class for me on epidemiology. There were about two hundred students in the lecture theatre and I went in the back door to catch the end of her lecture. There she was, waving her crutches in the air and hopping around the lecture theatre. At one stage she used her crutch as a pointer for the large screen and I could see the students were amused at her antics. She was a confident public speaker and there was a presence about her that filled the room. It was moments like these that would superimpose on how I saw her body and I think that is what she saw in my face—a sadness as I recalled the past in terms of the present.

Often nurses do not know the history of the people they care for and it is the family who reflect the grief and sadness of a time when their loved one was well. When I worked in one particular aged care setting the nurses had photographs and some stories of the residents in their rooms for people to share. One elderly man that I cared for was lying in the fetal position and did not speak or move. The photographs of him during his life and only a˙few months before he became so ill had an enormous impact on me. I was more easily able to relate to his family and their grief and it gave me something to talk about with this man—the story that the photographs revealed. Once, when MR was at home in between hospital admissions, she put her skis near her bed. For anyone who visited her they could not escape confronting MR's past, when she was fit and healthy, when they looked at the skis. I had looked at her feet twisted with foot drop and tried to imagine them in the binders, holding up her sturdy frame as she skied down slopes of snow.

MR: Not only has my illness changed the way that I look but I'm now pale from lack of sunlight and from being ill. I use to spend summers outdoors without protection despite the skin cancer scare. I enjoyed being tanned. Now my father calls me Casper. I never wore makeup other than lipstick occasionally for a special occasion. Now I wouldn't ask the nurses to put any on me. I think putting on makeup is a private and personal thing. If I wanted to put on makeup then I guess I would ask a friend.

When I am washed I am touched all over my body. I switch off from this as well because I reserve touching for those I love. I wonder if the nurses consider that I am a person when they touch me.

It would seem that MR has alienated herself from the nurses perhaps in order to cope with what they have to do with her. This probably began when so many different nurses came into intimate contact with such a private person every day. MR is ensuring that there is a certain distance between her and the nurses and this probably gives her a sense of privacy.

THE BALD HEAD

MR: My hair is very different now and not by choice. In 1994 my hair fell out. I was devastated as clumps fell out and adorned my pillow. It came out in handfuls when it was washed. The last straw was when my doctor commented on my mangy hair. It was worse while it was falling out to when I was completely bald. I am lucky because I think my face suited having no hair. My friends would call me Sinead O'Connor or Sigourney Weaver. Friends would say that it doesn't matter what you look like—well that's OK if it is not you. For me it was one more thing that I lost control of.

Having no hair is a signal to society that you are sick and maybe you might have cancer. I might deny my body but I do care how I look. Eventually and very slowly my hair has grown back. Now the problem is that lying all day on a pillow my hair gets matted and knotted. I only have it washed every two or three weeks due to the difficulty in bathing me. This, I felt, left me with no choice other than to shave it off except the hair on the very top. It's not what I would choose but it gives me some control. I have a friend who shaves my hair and she puts colour in the remaining hair which makes me feel much better.

Madjar (1997, p. 60) drawing on the work of Merleau-Ponty (1962) tells us 'the embodied knowing of one's own illness can be powerful in demonstrating the facticity of our corporeal existence, and the frailty and finitude of the only body through which each of us is able to live a life'. Madjar (1997, p. 60) further describes how people who are ill sometimes cannot see a way of regaining 'the habitual body' and that they need to see a way of moving towards a better future. She tells the stories of people who are alienated and repulsed by their ill bodies and says that hope is also an embodied existence. Although MR's descriptions of herself at this time are poignantly filled with grief of a body lost, she still nonetheless was hopeful that a diagnosis, treatment and recovery would propel her into a future she could still imagine. I believe that this explains, if only partially, how she is able to sustain such a terrifying existence. Somehow MR has been able to project her feelings of hope to all of her friends and family which assists us to cope with our despair.

MR: When I am in bed I feel the least pain so this is where I have spent 99 per cent of my time over the last few years. Being turned side to side represents the rare occasions when I get touched by other people. Yet I don't really see it as human contact—it is more a necessity. Turning me from side to side causes me severe pain. I am not the sort of person to writhe moaning and groaning in pain. It is not my way—I just retreat into my head. I have to cope. Maybe nurses don't realise I am in pain but they have always given me analgesics and now they give me morphine—so I wonder why they think I take that.

Madjar (1997, p. 63) argues that 'pain silences and actively destroys language, one of the culturally learned ways of being in the world with others'. As a phenomenon, Scarry (1985 in Madjar 1997, p. 62) states that pain 'more than any other phenomenon, resists objectification in language'. MR would rarely talk of her pain. There is a suspicion by others that if you have lost the sensation of your body then pain would be minimal or absent.

At the time when MR was seen as basic nursing care waiting for a diagnosis, the nurses would ask her if she wanted anything for pain when they gave out the drugs. It was only then that she was given analgesics—pain was not a subject that she or the nurses initiated a conversation about.

MR: I worry that there are many people out there without a nursing education caring for people with chronic illnesses. The changes in my health such as in my skin, breathing, mobility, speech, etc have been very subtle. My major area of concern has always been my coccyx and the skin on my buttocks. While I like to be active in my care I can't see all of my skin so I have to rely upon nurses and their expertise to prevent my skin from breaking down. I have a friend who is a nurse and I ask her to carefully check to see if my skin is breaking down because it happens so fast. The other thing I worry about is my circulation and sensation. I need the nurses to notice the subtle changes in me that I may not.

Interestingly MR refers to the day to day changes in her health and body as subtle. While this may be the case day to day the subtle changes over time were profound. The doctors struggled with how MR changed depending on their current theory of a diagnosis. Her diagnosis at the time, whether it was asthma or muscle weakness for investigation determined what the doctors chose to see. Often the *subtle* changes in her body that would amount over time to her being unable to walk would go unnoticed. The next chapter explores how the doctors were reacting to the changes in her body.

8

LUNGS OR LEGS

AN ONTOLOGICAL CRISIS

MR's story is one of being ill told within a reductive framework of medical science which, so far, she does not contest. Throughout this story, as MR struggles to retain her identity, her despair and the harsh reality of the separation of her self into a mind and a body is revealed. Along with her struggle to be given a diagnosis to explain her muscle weakness, MR had to eventually face what can only be described as a major crisis in her 'being' (an ontological crisis). This was when the full extent of her muscle weakness was realised and she was ultimately dismissed by the medical and nursing staff because she did not have a diagnosis and pathology to explain her illness.

MR: The doctor continued to see me and one day he came and he was actually nice to me, whereas he had been distant and abstract before. I'd just had a shower and I was really tired and breathless. He asked me if I was tired from the shower. I said 'Everything makes me tired' and he goes, 'Oh, that's very interesting'. You know, it was sort of like he was starting to think again about the problem. And it was quite fortunate that I was sitting in the chair because he looked at my legs and he goes, 'Oh, look at your legs; they're very wasted'. He had never, not once, examined my legs; he had only been interested in my lungs. Anyway, I said 'Yes, they've been like that for a while now'. And I said, 'They went like this within a matter of days of me being in hospital'. I told him how I was someone who runs, who had quite muscly legs, and how they had become bloody sticks. He said 'Oh, that's strange'.

Then he took blood gases and did a vitalograph and started talking about my lungs. He had forgotten, I think, that I went beyond being an 'asthmatic'. Anyway, he went then and didn't mention my legs again.

What stands out in MR's story is the way that MR articulates how the doctor constructed her as lungs. The doctor had obviously only had conversations with MR about her lungs, never about her legs, and certainly never about her. Finally, by accident, the doctor was confronted by actually seeing her legs. For a moment, MR began a conversation that she had desperately waited for—only to be dismissed as lungs again. As MR says he had forgotten that she went beyond being an asthmatic. This confusion, in her being either lungs or legs exemplifies 'how people are understood to be separated from their bodies, their world and those around them' (Parker 1991a, p. 295). MR's body is an object to her and others because of the Cartesian understandings of what it means to have a body within our culture.

Sacks (1984, p. 73) describes a similar experience to MR of how, when he mentioned to the doctor that he had lost sensation in his legs, he was ignored. He wondered what sort of doctor this man was, for clearly he had not heard him. MR, like Sacks (1984, p. 73) was totally frustrated in being cast in the 'know nothing' role of a patient. The doctor had given Sacks no opportunity to discuss his leg by saying 'No problems then, I take it'? Sacks had looked to the nurse for support but she did not speak. He said that he started to stammer when he told the doctor of his concerns (Sacks 1984, p. 72).

If Sacks, a respected doctor and a man, had difficulty telling the doctor about his loss of sensation in his leg, then perhaps we can understand MR's silence. While Sacks did speak, he was only able to stammer. Doctors, more so than nurses, meet the people they are caring for as patients, not as people, individuals with histories that are not only medical histories. The roles of doctor, nurse and patient are discursively created within a medical context and they then act to constrain, limit and contain what is said to each other within this predefined context. MR told the doctor that her legs had been strong and healthy before she became ill. In a sense she offered something of her history for the doctor to compare with what he now saw. The doctor ignored the cues—he was only there to examine her lungs.

Recently, a student of mine wrote a narrative about a similar situation. The person she was caring for asked her to tell the doctors of some of her concerns when they came on the round. The registered nurse, with the student, had said to her, *'They have to learn to speak up for themselves'*. We had quite a discussion analysing and theorising the notion of 'speaking up' in a hospital, especially when you are a patient, dressed in pyjamas, lying in a bed with other people listening to your conversation.

SCIENCE AND NOTHINGNESS

Sacks (1984, p. 77) describes being a patient as a point where he entered 'nothingness and limbo'. As the organic foundation of reality was removed from his life, he talks of falling into a hole:

> This would be tolerable, or more tolerable, if it could be communicated to others, and become a subject of understanding and sympathy—like grief. This was denied me when the surgeon said 'Nothing', so that I was thrown into the further hell—the hell of communication denied. (Sacks 1984, p. 77)

As Sacks later reflected, 'science and reason could not talk of "nothingness"' (Sacks 1984, p. 81). MR, too, seemed to turn inward as communication with medical science was denied her. Sacks (1984, p. 79) is very descriptive about this time when he was ill. He uses such terms as 'fallen off the map, out of time, inward and secret despair, a deadly inner silence' and comments on the humility he experienced when he could no longer equate himself with 'the active, masculine, ordering self' he says he equated with his science (1984, p. 79). I believe that it is this inward journey that ill people experience that brings them to the realisation of how alone they actually are. Many, such as Sacks, turn to religion for the comfort and security that they are not able to find in the people around them. MR is not religious but she silently held on to her belief that eventually doctors would find out what was wrong with her and 'make her better'.

MR: As my neuropathy overtook my body I needed lots more medications. I still take my asthma medication. In fact I am a demanding patient when it comes to asthma medications. Basically I am very frightened that I will have a serious asthma attack that will be life-threatening. It has been very difficult for nurses to understand my fear. What I mean is doctors always talk of decreasing my asthma medication. I have convinced myself that I might die if they do so. And as the drugs get decreased I think they don't care about me. I know that this is not true but remembering how I first became ill it's what I believe. Maybe I don't need all of the asthma medications but I want to feel safe and in control of my breathing.

MR equates the interest in her lungs and the medications she is given with care. After her experiences it would be reasonable to assume that if she was able to reduce the asthma medications it may be difficult to convince anyone that she needed them again or, indeed, that she was a person who had asthma at all. At times, when MR reflects on becoming ill it was directly related to her experiences of not being able to breathe.

MR: I imagine dying with asthma—fighting for every last breath. I have a real phobia of being unable to breathe and dying. The doctors have been quite insensitive when I explain my fear. In the initial stages of my illness breathing was the problem and I had been ventilated. I couldn't even sleep for fear that I would stop breathing and die. I never want to be on a ventilator again.

MR is confused about how doctors viewed her illness. She reminds us that breathing was of so much concern to the doctors that she was ventilated in ICU so that she could breathe.

MR: I tried to accept that I could not reclaim my body and I tried to think about being chronically ill. I needed to accept that I was no longer a physical being but I don't feel any less of a person because I feel disembodied.

As she began to experience being disembodied MR said little to the nurses or to the doctors as she continued to spiral on her inward journey. Cixous (in Minh-Ha 1991) who took seriously 'writing the body' and thereby made explicit links between power, discourse and the body, had the following words to say about the silence that inhabits women's writings. These thoughts have particular relevance to how I perceive the silencing of MR through her experiences of embodiment:

... I who had been nothing but the expression of hope in a language which had become extinct, no-one spoke to me any more, not spoken myself I abandoned myself, I didn't believe myself any more, my voice was dying in my throat, silence submerged it, I no longer heard anything but the silence. (Cixous in Minh-Ha 1991, p. 138)

MR: Eventually I stopped asking the doctors what was going on. I was sick of being treated as if I didn't know anything.

MR's whole way of being was gradually changing and I began to notice subtle changes in the way nurses routinely seemed to accept taking over more and more of her body care. Lawler (1991, p. 158) comments on how nurses can create an 'environment of permission' that normalises an ill person's experience but in this instance it was not helpful for MR. For the nurses it was business as usual as if this young woman, now in a quadriplegic state, was invisible to them. For MR it was confusing for the nurses to treat her experiences as 'normal'. She was facing losing the function of her entire body and so she desperately needed to talk with the people who cared for her about what was happening to her. Maybe then she could have discussed with them what it actually felt like.

BEING IN PAIN

Another issue that contributed to MR's silence was her pain.

MR: The pain that I experience permeates my every waking moment and even disturbs my sleep. It is strong and deep, penetrating, with an almost burning quality. It affects mainly my legs and back, but there are a few parts of my body that do not hurt. I am very unaware of my body except for the pain which does remind me of its existence in a very cruel way. I can hardly cope with my pain. Pain and tiredness dominate my life. Pain is very difficult to explain to other people, especially doctors. I understand that it can not be measured like other clinical signs and symptoms but that then becomes the problem.

  I prefer to lie quietly with my pain. The reason why I say 'my pain' is that it is my pain. Pain is so personal and difficult to explain. I don't think doctors like it because they have to rely on what the patient is

telling them. I once had to say to my doctor at the time, hey, this pain is so bad I want to die, before he would take it seriously.
Does it really matter if I get addicted to morphine? To be fair, for a long time my pain was never investigated properly. In desperation, I asked if I could see a pain specialist. I was already on slow release morphine for break-through pain. It seemed that the pain specialists could offer nothing further since my pain is of neuropathic origin. I just have to cope with ever-worsening pain.

Nothing about MR's way of being was untouched as everything about her was forced to change. No longer able to do anything for herself, in fact she could only talk, MR lay motionless.

LOSING SENSATION

MR: I began to lose the sensation of my legs, arms and hands, and the nurses and attendants turned me every two hours. I had to have a catheter; I hated that. If the nurses moved me and I couldn't see my legs, I had no idea where they were in the bed. I remember I asked you once to check on my legs and you found them stuck in the bed rails. I felt as if they were not connected to me.

When MR asked me to check on her legs I was initially confronted by the request. As I have discussed I rarely touched MR and she was asking me to look under the bedding that concealed her body. I pulled back the covers—she was very twisted and her legs were stuck in between the bed rails. As I freed her legs I noticed how her feet were like blocks of ice and she had red marks on them from their being wedged against the bed rails. While I had the covers back I asked MR about her legs and before I knew it, I found that I was examining her body. I tested her sensation, checked her circulation, and began to see how much movement she had. As I touched and explored her body she indicated that she could not feel any part of her legs. After covering her up we talked about the terrifying experience of losing sensation.

As MR lost sensation in her legs she began to struggle to conceive of her legs as part of her embodiment. Sacks (1984, p. 49) tells of his experiences of not 'knowing his leg'. As he lost the feeling for his leg he described his leg as 'foreign' to his body. He discusses how this felt:

> I turned at once to my leg, with a keen, startled and almost fierce attention. And in that instant, I no longer knew it. In that instant, that very first encounter, *I knew not my leg*. It was utterly strange, not-mine, unfamiliar. I gazed upon it with absolute non-recognition. (Sacks 1984, p. 47)

The loss of connectedness between MR and her legs brought about a further dissolution of reality for her. The actual sensation of not having legs was somewhat metaphysical as it could not be explained scientifically.

MR: It was really weird when I lost the sensation in my legs because I had no idea where they were in the bed. I wondered if I had a disturbance of proprioception because the paraesthesia and muscle paralysis could not be explained by any of the doctors.

Once again MR tries to explain the lost sensation in her legs scientifically. She asked me on another occasion to look to see if her legs were in a good position in the bed. This gave me another opportunity to touch and look at her legs again. As I repositioned her legs MR asked me to test her circulation and sensation responses again and it was awful as I waited for her to tell me she could feel the difference between sharp and dull pressure upon her skin, but she said nothing. I inspected her legs and massaged her feet for a while. It was in that moment, standing there with MR, confronted with her body, that I felt overwhelmingly sad and perhaps guilty that I had not massaged or exercised her legs before. I realised how I had struggled with being her friend and a nurse in a hospital where everyone knew me, and how this had silenced me into being the 'docile' visitor. That day as I massaged her feet I was scared by the cold unresponsive flesh that my hands touched. I could still feel the memory of her body in my sadness long after I left the hospital.

THE CATHETER

It was during this time that MR was to experience requiring even more assistance from the nurses. The details of her daily life were more and more exposed to others as she grew weaker. In particular, as she mentions, she had to contend with having a catheter.

MR: The catheter was awful and I suffered from many bladder and kidney infections. I had to have the catheter because I was unable to pass urine and at times I felt like my bladder would explode from the pressure. Being catheterised is an extremely private thing to have done. It's awful to lie there having your legs wide open. It certainly takes some adjusting. The nurses didn't seem embarrassed unless they made a mistake and missed the urethra and put it in my vagina because then they would have to start again.

I have noticed a whole range of reactions from women when I have catheterised them. Some have totally detached themselves from the procedure saying to me *'Do what you have to'*, or *'Just make it quick and tell me when you are finished'*, while others have been really involved in what I was doing. The first time I ever catheterised a woman, I took the trolley in with all of the equipment and the procedure manual on the bottom of the trolley. I had already practised the procedure on a plastic dummy and was quite confident that I could manage.

However, I do remember a moment of panic before I began. The nurse had told me that many new nurses 'put the catheter in the wrong hole'. I wondered how this might happen and hoped that I would recognise the 'right hole'. The woman was nothing like the plastic dummy and indeed it was with great relief that I did manage. It was a procedure that I learned as a recipe but the art to this procedure was not included in the book. The manual stated clearly to 'Prepare the patient' but this meant to screen the bed, remove the bedding and cover the top half of the woman. It took me quite a while before I believe that I managed the person, the procedure and myself.

Lawler (1991, p. 142) argues that nurses must learn to manage their own embarrassment to convey to the patient that they are not embarrassed or uncomfortable. She furthers argues that a 'crucial element in the management of embarrassment' occurs if nurses have 'a sense of purpose associated with having to perform particular nursing acts' (Lawler 1991, pp. 142, 143). I, like the nurses in Lawler's (1991, p. 142) study, have no recollection of being taught how to manage my own embarrassment.

THE ONLY 'PRIVATE AREA'

MR: Another private thing was if I menstruated. The nurses were offering to put the tampons in but I just couldn't let them. There was no way that I could allow this as it was just too personal. The nurses themselves didn't seem to understand why I wouldn't let them help me but I think that I needed to keep one area private. Menstruating was the one thing about care that really I didn't like others looking after. I was always worried that I would end up in a pool of blood and I felt that it was just too embarrassing to ask for help.

Emily Martin (1987, p. 92) argues that how women regard menstruation depends upon 'whether they have learned and adopted the medical model and the general cultural model or whether they have developed other kinds of models'. The general cultural view that menstruation is 'dirty' or a 'hassle' is a view that most women are aware of. Martin (1987, p. 93) found that women expressed that they regarded dealing with menstruation as a very private matter that no one else should see. MR expresses precisely these same sentiments.

Women usually find private places such as bathrooms and toilets to deal with menstrual blood but MR was confined to her public bed in a hospital. Her privacy was even more compromised because she either had to use a pad or take up the offers of the nurses to use a tampon. MR describes keeping one place, her vagina, as private as she could. She did not want the nurses to assist her with a tampon because it signalled that she had nothing left that was private. The nurses, on the other hand, would have offered to help her with tampons to spare her using pads so it would be more private for her but this offer somehow made her menstruation more explicit.

MR: I'm glad that I no longer menstruate, so it's no longer an issue.

Recently MR and I were discussing menstruation again and, she reiterated what a relief it is not to menstruate because she can maintain some privacy and dignity. However, most women in Martin's (1987) study, linked menstruation with being a woman and having children. MR is reminded by the absence of menstruation, every month, that her body has changed.

9

BEING 'A PSYCH CONSULT'

IS THE ILLNESS 'REAL'?

In the previous chapters MR has constructed herself as a head and the doctors have constructed her as lungs; then for a brief moment they shifted their attention to her legs. However because there was still no pathology to fix the doctors' interest on any specific part of her body, they also turned their attention to her head.

MR: One day the doctor came to see me and mentioned my legs again. He said, 'Have you walked yet?' Surely it was obvious I couldn't move, let alone walk. Then he said, 'We are not sure what is going on,' and they all started to think it was psychogenic. I was devastated.

And this is when the nurses started to be different. I think their attitude to me was that I was a bit of a bother, because they had to do all these things with me. I remember how they made me sit out of bed in that chair; and I remember one day I slipped out and got caught in the hole between the chair and the footrest—it was one of those Jason Recliners. I was stuck there forever, without a buzzer. When the nurses came in I yelled and swore at them so they rushed and got the attendants to get me out. I have never seen them move so fast. I thought how horrible they were to me, only . . . you know . . . now it doesn't seem so bad. But I was in that hole for an hour.

This account from MR tells of how frustrated she had begun to feel. It must have been very strange to be asked by the doctor if she had walked yet. It was obvious, especially to those who cared for her, that she was unable to move let alone walk. In asking the question *'Have you walked yet?'* the doctor was dismissing MR because he implied that MR could walk if she wanted to. He then dismissed MR yet again by saying that they, the medical profession, could not explain MR's condition. As soon as he said psychosomatic, MR was re-positioned as having a condition, rather than an illness, where there was no disease and no diagnosis. It was not possible then for MR to be afforded an illness that could be recognised as a 'real' illness.

Once the doctors had implied to MR that her illness may not be real she deteriorated rapidly. I found the experience of watching her get weaker almost by the hour very frightening. The medical staff, once again, reacted to her decline by re-investigating every system they could. Soon she had a new site of invasion on her body: bruises from venipuncture, sutures from muscle biopsies and red marks from electrodes. She was referred from specialist to specialist including all of the allied health professionals. With every day, as she waited for a diagnosis, MR seemed to slip further into her illness. She lost more weight and muscle tone to the point where her skin seemed to drape itself in folds around her bones. Once again all of the tests failed to reveal a diagnosis.

MR: You know, I didn't have anything to eat for weeks and I was becoming bruised all over from having blood taken every day. There was one day that they took blood from me ten times. I was very sick. I couldn't swallow or move very well and the nurses had to do nearly everything for me. I even had a lumbar puncture, and then I had really bad headaches as well.

CARING FOR A DIAGNOSIS

Apart from the sensory losses that MR was experiencing in her arms and legs there was sometimes the problem of her being unable to swallow. At times she even seemed to gag on her own saliva. One evening when I visited MR I was to walk into her room when she was choking. There was a nurse with her, but I was concerned to notice that she seemed to be ignoring the choking. The nurse was calmly saying, 'Nice deep breaths, MR'. I was scared because this was what MR had done on our walk and she had the same distressed look. I asked the nurse if she could use the sucker but she said she had to go and get something and she left the room. For a few moments I was left with a very blue and petrified MR. When the nurse finally came back, she casually and reluctantly used the sucker and MR improved slightly. I sensed that there was a changed attitude in all of the nurses on the ward who now acted differently.

This particular nurse, who sensed my shock, took me aside and told me that all of the tests were negative and that MR was for a psych consult. I felt absolute despair and disappointment with the nurse's attitude and found myself feeling there was nothing to say to her. From that time on I do not believe that MR was ever cared for consistently in the same way again. Once the doctors had written *For a psych consult* in her history, there appeared to be an impact upon some of the nurses and the care that they gave to MR. The blurred boundaries of the body and the mind were now clearly demarcated. A rupture had occurred with the reductionist mind-body split, enforced and reinforced by medical discourse. I was as guilty as everyone else in that while we were waiting for a diagnosis, we had let MR's whole way of being slip away.

MR: The nurses stopped caring for me from the time a doctor wrote in my history *For a psych consult*. The whole manner of the nurses towards me changed yet none of them ever discussed this issue with me. I was left for long periods of time and I was really frightened and lonely. I imagined that during handover the psych consult bit was always being discussed about me, but little else. Before this time the nurses used to talk with me about my medical condition but then they started to talk with me about my social status, like my family and what I like to do. This worried me because then it was up to me to remember what was happening to me medically so I could tell someone. I would worry about getting an infection (and I often did) in my bladder or lungs. I might be really ill by the time anyone noticed and the antibiotics might be given too late. In the end the worry was too much—it became so hard.

No longer considered an asthmatic, MR was re-situated as someone who may have been responsible for her illness. When doctors appeared to give up by handing over MR to psychiatry it reinforced that the illness was not real and that her illness was all in her head.

According to Leder (1984, p. 40), to attribute the cause of an illness to be either in the body or the mind exposes the rigidity and the extremes of Cartesian dualism. The doctors could not diagnose an organic cause or disease process to explain MR's illness. They could not explain the illness through pathologising MR's body, so the alternative was to try to explain MR's illness through her mind.

HYSTERICAL OR MENTAL

Although MR never mentioned the notion of hysterical conversion reactions, the doctors most certainly had. Organic paralysis was observed by Freud to have neuro-anatomical patterns, while he argued that hysterical paralysis did not obey these patterns. According to Sacks (1984, p. 176), Freud saw these two forms of paralysis as either mental or physical and these were the working definitions that all doctors including psychiatrists came to use. The significance of this for MR was enormous because the medical profession believe that, if paralysis or anaesthesia cannot be explained anatomically through disease or trauma they must, 'by default be "hysterical" or "mental"' (Sacks 1984, p. 176). Sacks (1984, p. 177) argues that this disallows 'any investigation or understanding of *other* states' of paralysis and prevents any exploration of the neuropsychological disturbances of body-image and 'self'. MR's illness, paralysis, and the way she was or was not treated fit Sacks's observations. When Sacks was ill he realised that not even he, as a neurologist, could escape the rigid dualism of mind and body.

Dreyfus observes, in Foucault's 'Maladie Mentale et Personalite', the 1976 translation, that Foucault's aim was to 'show that mental pathology requires methods of analysis different from those of organic pathology and that it is only by an artifice of language that the same meaning can be attributed to "illnesses of the body" and illnesses of the mind' (Foucault in Dreyfus 1976, p. ix). It is interesting to note that Foucault examines the history of madness as a social and cultural construct. Foucault (1976, p. 63) asks 'how did our culture come to give mental illness the meaning of deviancy and to the patient a status that excludes him [sic]'. Even with some understanding of how this may have happened in the past it does not justify how, in 1998, society still ignores and hides behind the rhetoric of something referred to as mental health.

All of my undergraduate students undertake a subject known

as mental health. When they first enter the mental health practice world they are both scared and fearful of mental illness. They can all recall a story from within their own family or a family they know well that has shaped their beliefs of mental illness. They are scared of 'madness' and what that might mean. More than any other reason they are worried as to how they might talk with people living with mental illness. One student told my tutorial group how she went on a bus trip with some people who live with a mental illness. She described hiding behind dark sunglasses crouching down in her seat on the bus in case anyone should recognise her. 'How would people know I was the student and they were the patients?' she asked.

So entrenched is the fear of mental illness in society that the students' own personal fear of being a 'psych' patient stays with them. They argue that despite their ability to critique and understand how society constructs something called mental illness there is a fear of that very construction being applied to them. I have a friend who often tells me about 'his year on the couch' as he puts it. I am always impressed with the way that he includes this aspect of his life in the stories that he chooses to tell about himself. He reminds me of many Americans, almost proud to have an analyst, but this was not a psychologist but a psychiatrist that he saw. I know that I would resist telling people if I had seen a psychiatrist because I know that I would fear being labelled as having a psych history. Imagine being permanently under surveillance for any future signs of 'abnormality' by friends and family. The society that we live in does not easily accommodate difference—and people with mental illness are socially constructed as different—and thus they are marginalised.

RECOGNISING THE 'SELF' IN THE REJECTED BODY

Foucault (1976, p. 62) said that American psychologists examined illness:

> ... from both a negative and possible point of view. It is negative, since illness is defined in relation to an average, a norm, a 'pattern', and since the whole essence of the pathological resides within this departure: illness it seems, is marginal by nature and relative to a culture only insofar as it is a form of behaviour that is not integrated by that culture.

He further argued that 'our society does not wish to recognise itself in the ill individual whom it rejects or locks up' (Foucault 1976, p. 63).

This is the fear to which I refer—that of recognising the self in the rejected body. This same fear is expressed through the nurses' behaviour with MR after she was referred to the psychiatrist.

MR: In my single isolation room it was easy for the nurses to avoid me. It would have not been so easy to be ignored in a shared room. Out of sight out of mind. The nurses only saw me when they had to. I think it was more comfortable for them not to see me. It must have been the short straw for the nurse who was allocated to look after me. Interestingly I never saw a psychiatrist during this time.

Once the doctors had written in MR's history 'For a psych consult' they had, in some sense, assigned MR a provisional diagnosis. According to Pilgrim and Treacher (1992 in Horsfall 1997, p. 179), 'the medical–psychiatric way of looking at these human experiences is hegemonic amongst the majority of nurses and other health workers'. She further argues that 'one does not find the (whole) body in the mental health nursing texts, neither can one find the (whole) mind, let alone a person' (Horsfall 1997, p. 184). The nurses who cared for MR were probably not only fearful of her illness and what it might represent to them but also were displaced by the doctors' suggested psych consult.

I can remember caring for someone on a surgical ward with abdominal pain when they were subsequently diagnosed as having anorexia. The nurses would all say at handover that this patient should not be on our ward because there was nothing we could do for them. Yet, when the nurses had believed that the same person had nausea and was an 'abdominal pain for investigation' they knew just what to do. The nurses may have avoided MR, as she suggests, but perhaps they were initially avoiding confronting how they might actually care for her. From speaking to some of the nurses at the time there seemed to be a feeling that they had been led astray by the doctors because they had believed MR 'really' was paralysed and now they were confused that it may not be 'real'. Others even thought that if they were out of the room that she could probably move, while a few believed that the doctors were wrong and that she had an illness that had been altogether missed.

GUILTY UNTIL INNOCENT

MR: Dealing with the prejudices of being labelled as having a problem in my head has been soul destroying in itself. I thought there was something seriously wrong with me, yet I was treated like a loony! How was I supposed to deal with my body? I do have something called psychotherapy now and I see that as an integral component of my treatment but not as treating a cause of my illness. Not at any time, or any time since it was written in my history, have I entertained the notion that my condition was all in my head, psychosomatic, an hysterical conversion or anything else, other than an organic disease. I was admitted into hospital with asthma and then I ended up like this. It was so easy to sweep me under the carpet and I was guilty until proven innocent.

MR tells us that she was not even given the same treatment as criminals who are presumably innocent until proven guilty. She knew that they had no proof, as it were, that her illness was psychosomatic. It is difficult to imagine what it must have been like to be so ill that you could not move and then not only to be blamed for the illness but also to be abandoned by medicine. MR has always believed that her illness is organic in origin. I, on the other hand, have tended to think about how she is now—not searching for reasons as to how she became ill. Of course, I can do this because I do not have to live out the illness or the consequences of the way an illness is described. Whether the origins of her illness are psychosomatic or organic, MR *is* an ill *person*. That she likens herself to a criminal is criminal in itself and an issue that medicine and nursing cannot afford to ignore. We will never move beyond Cartesian understandings of the body while the discipline of psychiatry claims the mind.

Foucault (1976, p. 64) traces the historical constitution of mental illness. He claims that in the seventeenth and eighteenth centuries there was not yet an obvious distinction between psychological and physical. In the nineteenth century 'madness ceased to be regarded as an overall phenomenon affecting, through the imagination and delusion, both body and soul' (Foucault 1976, p. 72). From that time on the phenomenon of mental illness has persisted and Foucault (1976, p. 76) argues that as a term 'mental illness is simply *alienated madness*, alienated in the psychology that it has itself made possible'.

When I started to think and read about madness and psychosomatic states I found a repeated and confusing theme in the literature. Many authors discuss the fact there are people with 'genuine' psychosomatic illnesses. There are also people who are wrongly diagnosed as having a psychosomatic illness when they have a 'genuine' illness that is pathological in origin. Does that mean then, that those who have a genuine psychosomatic state are imagining and responsible for their illness? If so, what do we really understand about this because to argue that an illness is genuine is to also imply that some people are not genuinely ill. I would suggest that to say a person has a genuine psychosomatic illness is to also say that they are not genuinely ill and that in fact they do not have a illness but a condition. It is a contradiction that is highly problematic.

Wendall (1996, p. 99) discusses research that reveals many people are wrongly diagnosed with a psychosomatic illness. She argues that when this happens the diagnosis is not based on 'positive evidence of psychological problems: it was a *default diagnosis for physical symptoms*' (Wendall 1996, p. 99). She further discusses that illness such as chronic fatigue immune dysfunction syndrome, became recognised as a legitimate illness after 1988 and, many people before that time were wrongly diagnosed (Wendall 1996, p. 99). Such stories are not uncommon, I have heard people with illnesses ranging from cancer to a vitamin deficiency telling their stories of being diagnosed as having a psychological condition only to later find that they were 'really' ill.

It is this rather grey area of medicine that I have serious concerns with. My main concern is that doctors do not seem to be able to say that they just do not know why some people become ill. They have not broadened their horizon sufficiently, as yet, to incorporate other disciplinary approaches to health and illness, for example sociology, medical anthropology and nursing. And society has an expectation of medicine to hold and know the 'truth' about bodies when they become ill.

Consider the educational experiences that doctors have. Even with some medical schools changing aspects of their curriculum, most courses are still confined and limited by being purely biomedical science. As I have discussed, science not only leaves out the person but also society and culture, politics, history, gender and so on. Perhaps we should acknowledge the limitations of medicine and encourage doctors to say, I do not know what is wrong with you. At the same time, as a society, I believe we have invested too much power in medicine and we have expectations of medicine that often contribute to our own demise. If we continue to treat doctors like gods instead of health professionals with limitations, nothing may ever change.

Wendall (1996) and others have written about their experiences of being wrongly diagnosed as having a psychosomatic illness. These stories have come to expression because these people experience that they themselves are personally responsible for their illness. They experience feelings of being legitimate when they eventually receive a diagnosis. With a diagnosis they are somehow freed to be ill. MR was in a sense made prisoner to the discursive myths that the term psychosomatic perpetuates.

MR: I was really worried when the staff stopped asking me about my physical body and they all seemed to stop looking for a disease any more. Now it was my social life that everyone wanted to know about. It felt to me like people had suddenly become nosy, after all they had never wanted to know about my past life before. If I choose to tell someone about me then that is my choice and not their right to know. I was deliberately vague in the details of the answers to the questions that they were asking me. I did not want to tell anyone anything unless it would affect the care that I was going to receive. It was just none of their business.

EXPRESSING ILLNESS

I deliberately avoid a discussion on the mind and the body here and the myth that the mind controls the body—mind over matter—because I believe that the real issues get lost in such a discussion. I agree with Frank (1991, p. 127) when he says that he believes the responsibility of the ill 'is not to get well but to express their illness well'. He says that 'perhaps someday we might understand more of how the mind affects the body' (Frank 1991, p. 126). I wonder—I like to think that we will understand more about people and their bodies.

What is sad is that MR tells us that up until now the nurses always talked with her about her body, usually in a mechanistic way—MR would have encouraged this. She did not have conversations about her actual experiences of embodiment. When the nurses focused on her social history asking her questions about her family MR was suspicious. This was because it seemed that the staff were searching for some trauma in her past to explain her condition. I know MR would not have told every nurse her history, in fact very few, but given the opportunity she would have appreciated talking about her body and her experiences of being ill in the same conversation.

MR: The hard thing was that I had to tell the nurses about my medical problems because they started to ignore all of that. This problem has continued until the present day. For example once I had surgery on my nasal cavities which resulted in a great deal of contusions and sniffing. A nurse looking after me asked me if I was getting the flu. It was obvious to me that they were oblivious as to what was happening to my body.

We have heard how MR had previously been searching for clues as to what was happening to her body when she thought that the doctors must be missing something. Now she voices her concern that, while they all focus on her social history, she might have to resume her detective work. She had been relying on nurses to do this 'detective' work for her so that they could tell her what was happening to her body (medically). When the nurse did not know that MR had left the ward for surgery she was convinced that they were oblivious to her body now and only aware of her mind.

BEING DEPRESSED

MR: A couple of years into my illness the stress of everything really got to me and I became very depressed. I couldn't concentrate and my feeling of overwhelming sadness took over. I was so sad that I could feel it physically as tightness in my chest. This was when I did see a psychiatrist and he became my sounding board and was helping me to grieve the loss of my life. He discussed antidepressants with me. He thought that the stress had led to a chemical imbalance in my brain and that I needed a six-month course of serotonin re-uptake inhibitors. Surprisingly, I found myself agreeing. Prior to my illness I was totally against psychiatrists and their drugs as I saw that there was a social stigma attached to submitting to such treatment. Now I can appreciate what psychiatry has to offer.

I'm sure that the way that MR's depression was explained to her as a 'chemical imbalance' influenced her decision to take antidepressants. It was a voice of science that she responded to. Horsfall

(1997, p. 181) refers to contemporary psychiatry and its relationship to neuro-anatomy, electrochemistry, and psycho-endocrinology. She argues that 'medical researchers seem to be determined that neurotransmitters are at the bottom of our most socially feared psychiatric disorders' (Horsfall 1997, p. 181). If this unfortunate trend continues it may eventually be possible to blame the body for that which the mind was previously blamed and all illnesses will be pathological in origin. That would leave psychology to deal with conditions and the mind.

MR was pleased to have someone to talk to. It is not flippant to suggest that it is a pity that other doctors had not talked with her. Frank (1990, p. 140) comments that Kleinman's remarks 'that it is possible to talk with patients, even those who are most distressed, about the actual experience of illness', can only be news to physicians. Ironically MR has now got a doctor for her mind, but not for her body, unless she gets an infection or her medications need reviewing.

Horsfall (1997, p. 178) discusses how 'depressions reveal certain socially stigmatised attitudes of mind and body'. She argues that the depressed body is stigmatised because 'the mind is faulty' (Horsfall 1997, p. 178). By this remark Horsfall is making explicit the way a depressed person is alienated from the material productive world because they are viewed as slow, unreliable and gloomy people (Horsfall 1997, p. 178). MR said to me, *'Well wouldn't you be depressed if you had endured what I have?'* We can all relate to depression where a cause can be identified. However, people are not supposed to stay depressed. They are supported for a certain period of time and then expected to 'get over it' or 'snap out of it'. I see the main problem for MR is that by isolating one aspect of her illness, depression, means that once again that is all that will be treated—the depression not her. This serves to fragment MR even further because depression, as a term, conceals rather than reveals experiences of people.

MR: So, of course, agreeing to see the psychiatrist just confirmed for everyone that I had a problem. I was scared that everyone would think I was loony. I hesitated telling people that I was seeing a psychiatrist. However, it never bothers me now. It has helped me so much. Within a couple of months of taking the medication and the therapy I felt better—the sadness dissipated, my sleeping patterns improved. I came off the medication at one point to see how I was, and I got flashbacks from being in ICU. Every time I tried to talk about my past I would get sad. I went back on the medication and I admit that I need it to keep my depression at bay. Certainly I am not ashamed of taking this drug. As my condition deteriorates there will certainly be many other drugs that I need.

If MR was taking any other drug such as an antibiotic she would not feel compelled to justify it. People do feel ashamed that they are taking a drug for the mind because in our culture it implies a sign of weakness and such treatments are viewed with suspicion. The antidepressant drugs appeared in medicine in the 1950s and Capra (1982, p. 128) suggests that the popularity of these drugs can be attributed to the fact that 'psychiatrists were able to control a variety of symptoms and behaviour patterns of psychotics'. While these drugs are successful for controlling symptoms they also successfully obscure the problem. If medicine is limited by a biomedical approach then this limitation is at the extreme in psychiatry. Capra in 1982 remarked 'the extension of the biomedical model to the treatment of mental disorders has been, on the whole, very unfortunate' (1982, p. 143). I would argue that little has changed since Capra made these remarks and that psychiatrists and other medical practitioners remain segregated from each other professionally (thereby maintaining a distance between mind and body)—which is why MR became a psych consult.

10

RE-INVESTING IN SCIENCE

THE ILLNESS AS 'IT'

I have argued that, initially, MR's body was colonised by medicine as an object for the intervention of experts. Then, similar to Sacks' (1991) comments, medicine abandoned her body as psychiatry prepared to colonise her mind as medical territory. At this point MR had no alternative other than to conceive herself as just a head because that was the way medicine and psychiatry also constructed her. She was not, however, prepared to become a psychiatric patient.

MR: So, some people didn't think that I was 'really ill' any more. The only people who looked to the future were the physiotherapists as they continued to work on my body. Some nurses tried to trick me into doing things such as move my legs or arms. They needed proof that '*it*' was in my head . . . I can't explain it; the nurses were just very different to me. Once when the nurse made me hold the toothbrush to clean my teeth my head fell in the sink—I nearly drowned. I knocked my head so many times because it was so floppy.

I was assigned to a primary nurse who used to insist trying to stand me up to transfer me by herself if I wanted to use the commode or have a shower. However, I was really too much for her. She used to have to drag me because I just couldn't help her. When she managed to finally get me on the commode chair I felt as if my head was going to explode . . . honestly I felt so sick, it was absolutely shocking. The pain was just horrible . . . it was really bad.

I had a nasogastric tube down now. God, I remember the trauma of that going down. I bled out of my nose and my mouth.

There was one occasion when I did feel connected to my primary nurse and this was when some concern was shown that I had an abnormal ECG. She had got really upset when they wanted to do tests on me. I think she cried. I said to her, 'Look, I know the doctors don't know what's going on with me; I don't understand all of this stuff either.' She admitted she was really worried. When I went for the tests, she actually came with me and, just for once, she was checking it all out for me, like she was really concerned about it . . . know what I mean?

The primary nurse tried to transfer MR alone because she may have believed that MR would eventually 'help herself'. On this particular ward the nursing staff had adapted something they referred to as 'primary nursing'. As far as I could make it out it was a rhetorical term and, while MR had a little more contact with one nurse that she referred to as her primary nurse, nothing else was any different than on any other ward.

MR was able to establish one very positive relationship with a nurse (Marie) during this time. If Marie was working she was often with her and always nearby. One day I sat while Marie washed MR and the empathy she had for her was so visible I could feel it. More importantly MR could feel it. What MR and I so admired about Marie was the way that she did not conceal her own fear or sadness in relation to what was happening to MR. MR was always less defensive and more relaxed if Marie was caring for her, so much so that years later I clearly remember the difference that Marie made to MR because they were the days that I saw MR smile.

MR refers to her unknown illness as 'it' when she says that the doctors and nurses needed proof that it was real. In the literature and in general conversation, it becomes apparent that illnesses with no known cause, that collectively become psychosomatic states, are described as 'it'. With a diagnosis, 'it' becomes the cancer, the fractured leg, the tumour, the gall stone, the kidney condition, the heart condition, the ulcer and so on. MR was devastated because, semantically, the doctors had transformed her illness to 'it' and the possibilities of reality became imaginary. MR who had become the innocent, passive patient awaiting a diagnosis had been transformed into the culpable (Kirmayer, in Benoist and Cathebras 1993, p. 862). She was culpable because now it was possible to blame MR for her own illness. Sontag (1990) has also written of this phenomenon.

> The widely held view that many or even most diseases are not 'really' physical but mental (more conservatively, 'psychosomatic') perpetuates the form of the miasmic theory—with its surplus of causality, surplus of meaning—in a new version that has been extremely successful in the twentieth century. (Sontag 1990, p. 131)

GETTING BACK THE OLD LIFE

MR: I gradually felt out of control and I started to have really bad headaches and at times I thought that my head was going to explode. I was floppy. I couldn't swallow properly, I wasn't getting any nutrition, my chest was hurting, I couldn't breathe properly, and I just didn't know what was going on. I thought they were going to let me die. I decided that I had to get out of there so I enlisted the help of my friend Sally in organising for me to be transferred to a Melbourne hospital. Even if a diagnosis could still not be found, I was convinced that with proper care and rehabilitation that I would get back to my old life. I am not sure what the hospital staff thought about me going to another hospital. Nothing was said to me. My doctor may have been glad that I was going to be someone else's responsibility.

MR was scared enough to completely re-think her situation. She helped organise her transfer to a large Melbourne hospital. For a week MR seemed to come into focus again. The doctors and nurses looked anxious because MR was re-situating herself again by giving up her body to another institution for scientific investigation. A doctor approached me about accompanying MR, but when the nursing staff learnt of this, they all said it should be one of them because they were caring for her. MR did not really care who accompanied her as long as she got there. Her last week on the ward was marked with many people coming to wish her well. After so long being ignored MR seemed to enjoy being acknowledged, even if only for a week.

MR: I flew on a commercial airline flight to Melbourne on December 4, 1992. I was harnessed into a special stretcher bed and suspended from the ceiling at the back of the plane. I took up nine normal seat spaces and my seat number on the boarding pass said 'bed'. When I got to Melbourne there was some sort of dispute over who was responsible to get me off the plane. Eventually the catering lift was used and off I went in the ambulance to hospital.

I was relieved to go to the other hospital. It was a chance, I thought, to find out what was going on and get better. It was good; I sort of felt like I was going to be in safer medical hands. It was a long day but finally I was put into bed four, in a room where no-one, except me, spoke English. It was quite different. This was going to be my medical salvation. They chucked me in a bed and I waited for what seemed like ages for my new specialist team to do a round. The nurses came along and said 'In your own words, why are you here?' and I sort of said 'To have some tests and find out what's going on'. I wanted the latest—really good physios and equipment. I had it in my mind they could come up with some sort of idea of what was wrong with me medically; a medical box.

Anyway he came, the specialist, and he ordered a barrage of tests covering everything: bloods, lumbar punctures, nerve conduction studies, nerve velocity studies, an EMG, an MRI . . . that sort of thing. I spent hours having tests done. I was extremely floppy (I weighed 40 kg) and they fixed me up with a neck brace. The physios worked on me twice a day. I was still having swallowing problems . . . nausea and stuff. My poor gut. That had been a feature the whole time but they never considered that, never really. It's the same sort of thing that they really can't concentrate on more than one thing at a time.

MR had gradually lost confidence in the local doctors and the nurses, but not in science—that is why she changed hospitals. There was also the honeymoon period that she could enjoy again. Interestingly the nurse admitting MR asks her to use her own words to explain why she is in hospital. This implies that the words of a person are usually not their own once they are in hospital, unless they are given permission. On many nursing admission forms one section states 'In the patient's own words'. MR who is comfortable with, and uses complex medical language, puts her reasons for being in hospital into lay language to accommodate and to avoid confronting the nurse.

MR uses the metaphor of 'medical salvation', through which science and religion seem to fuse, implying she hopes to be saved.

While she still wanted a diagnosis, or medical box, she continued to view psychiatry with suspicion. Her poor gut that she refers to had always been a problem to her and she remarks that during her entire illness doctors only seemed to be able to concentrate on one thing at a time instead of working with all of the complex problems that she now had.

AN 'INTERESTING CASE'

MR: I had many investigations and eventually they said, 'We're not really sure what it is'. So they asked me all these questions: I was a very interesting case—very interesting, they said. They sent a psychiatrist to see me; they said everyone in neurology sees one. The doctor said many people with neurology problems can't be diagnosed—like 65 per cent of them, which was comforting to hear. I mean, it should not really matter whether they put you into a medical box, or not—but we are all brought up to believe you should be put in one. I didn't like the psychiatrist; I used to pretend to be asleep when she came. In the end she gave up coming. I became incredibly wasted, you know; I couldn't move to save my life.

Because it was explained that everyone in neurology sees a psychiatrist, MR did not feel as though she was being cast aside by the neurologists so she agreed to see one. Relieved with the doctors' interest in her as a medical case again, MR had been told that they may not be able to diagnose her. MR expresses how the notion of being brought up to believe that people who are ill must have a medical box has dominated her illness experience. MR infers that while she understands the problems with medical boxes, if you are not medicalised through a diagnosis, then you are alienated and marginalised from what most people understand about being ill.

MR: The 'ultimate' (and I say this sarcastically) experience for me was when they presented me at a grand round for the whole hospital. I had to be there. I was famous for a day—they were all extremely interested. I was wheeled in on the trolley.

THE GRAND ROUND

MR explained to me that she was pleased about the grand round idea because she was to be given an opportunity to have many medical people in the one space so that their collective knowledge could come together. This grand round was a gathering of doctors in a lecture theatre, rather than at the bedside, and MR was pleased that her 'case' had been selected for presentation. This signalled to her that the doctors were prepared to discuss her medical history and that they were not entirely sure what was wrong with her.

MR: The consultant said to me, 'We'd like to present your case at the grand round, because '*it*' is such an interesting case and your diagnosis, while there are some aspects of it we know (we can say you've got such and such, and such and such), there are some inexplicable factors which we think would benefit from a grand round'. And he was quite good really because he was appreciative of my medical background, and he knew some things about me. He knew I had been an asthmatic and all of that stuff; he was quite nice. Anyway, I had no idea I had to be there in person, and in the morning all these nurses were getting me washed and dressed. The charge nurse came and told them to make sure I was ready for the grand round. Then I went on a huge epic journey.

Note the 'it' in the quote from MR. The illness, that is the interesting case, it, was going to be presented at the grand round, housed in the body of MR. MR recalls that the doctor was quite good because he acknowledged that she has a bioscientific background and because he knew things about her. And what of the nurses all bustling around MR? Even the charge nurse visited her to hurry things along. I recall my own experiences of getting people ready for bedside grand rounds. Part of the rush is fear of the person not being in bed for the doctors, or that the ward might have the telltale signs of body care, such as a bowl still out or an unfortunate odour in the air. This reveals the ways that nurses are disciplined in institutions and the relationship that nursing has to medicine. MR and the nurses endorse the exercise of power by medicine by such behaviour.

MR did not usually have several nurses as well as the charge nurse concerned about her body care. She was being groomed for a special occasion. The practices and language of MR and the nurses positioned them as 'other' to medicine as they were silenced, subjugated, and marginalised. Walker (1993, p. 105) argues that 'nurses constitute the colonised "other", as *both a cause and an effect* of something of the conditions of their existence'. The doctor, closest to science, silently and effectively exercises power through the grand round, a time of medical worship. For one day MR was no longer ignored, as her body was to be investigated, objectively, at the grand round.

MR: I was wheeled to the grand round by the resident doctor and the charge nurse. The registrar came and got me and I couldn't believe the number of people in the lecture theatre. The consultant spoke about me as if I was not there or not a person anyway. At one stage he said 'Listen to the voice', and I had to speak. He demonstrated how I had no reflexes. I had to leave when they discussed me. The registrar told me I had done well. Anyway, eventually they said to me, 'We're not sure what you have got'.

I had every bloody medical specialist team in that hospital to visit me; you name it they came around to see me. They'd ask me had I ever been bitten by a tick, or had I ever been to Germany. No-one was intimating psychosomatic . . . well, not to me anyway. No one was ever like they were to me in the other hospital. I was interesting, but they never found a diagnosis; so in the end they decided to send me to a big rehabilitation hospital.

The resident doctor and the charge nurse accompanied MR to the lecture theatre, then the registrar wheeled her in for the consultant who talked about her. I find fascinating the way that she travelled through the hierarchy of medicine to get to the grand round. The charge nurse is positioned with the resident, which explains her interest in assisting MR to be ready for the round.

MR left this hospital having confronted some of the implications of the chronicity of her illness experience. She was obviously disappointed that she had no diagnosis, and that she had not improved; but she left believing that she was an interesting case and that her illness was not psychosomatic—and therefore not in her mind. I think that this point is very important because MR was able to regain a certain sense of her self by feeling legitimate again. She was given back a position she was more comfortable to be in. MR had succeeded, at least for a while, in resisting being abandoned to the struggle of being 'just a head'.

CONFRONTING THE BODY

MR: In the rehab hospital I got a bed beside a large picture window with a view out over the suburbs, which I thought was a good sign. Different nurses came in to say hello and then they said they would give me a shower as I told them it had been three weeks since the last one. Two nurses put on gumboots and plastic aprons. I was very confronted by my body, I had not looked at it for weeks. Did that body belong to me? The care that the nurses took that day was in stark contrast to how I had been treated in those early days. I really enjoyed having that shower and the nurses usually ended up having one as well.

Also I met another patient who explained to me the whole system of the ward. She told me who to avoid and the do's and don'ts and she offered me words of encouragement.

The thing that was hard was to tell my story again and again, over and over.

MR had not looked at her body because she had been bathed in the bed. As I have said before, being naked in the shower was confronting for her because she actually saw her body. While she was covered most of the time, and since she could not feel her body, she was usually able to sustain a certain detachment from her body.

MR: I was introduced to the commode chair and I nearly passed out with pain as my de-fleshed bones made contact with the unyielding metal and plastic. I wondered who designed such equipment. Then my therapy started. Well . . . from the sublime to the ridiculous! I started at 9.00 a.m. and I had an hour for lunch then went again until 4.00 p.m. I did improve a little in rehab but never fast enough. Every day I was tied to what I called the Hannibal Lecter table, so that I could be vertical. My neck would hurt and I would feel faint and I remember my arms and hands would go purple. My body seemed so foreign to me and very tired and painful.

Everything about the way MR had been previously cared for had changed. All of her effort now became focused on her body and on moving. While this was exactly what she had wanted, she had been so inactive for so long it came as quite a shock to her.

THE HONEYMOON WAS OVER

MR: Soon the honeymoon period was over and the staff began to show their frustration as I did not seem to improve much, and I know that I became stubborn. My upper arms got stronger, but that's about all. Falling was my biggest problem—I fell out of my chair, especially in the shower. Once I fell in the shower while the nurse had gone off for a moment. It was only that another patient noticed all the water running out of the shower that I was found when I was. A lot of the time the nurses and physiotherapists were hoping that I would make some effort to get up if I did fall. I really wanted to have hydrotherapy, but they said that I might drown so I never did.

It did not take long before, as MR says, she became 'stubborn' and the nurses became frustrated. Interwoven throughout MR's story of being in the rehabilitation hospital is her frustration. She remarks on the unspoken belief 'that she could move if she either had to or wanted to'. MR perceived that they expected her to move if the will and desire to move was stimulated in her. MR became stubborn; if she thought anyone was trying to trick her into moving, she would not even try. If MR had made some spontaneous movement what might that have signalled—perhaps that she had 'deliberately' not been moving?

The months passed with very little change despite all of the physiotherapy and MR began to worry about where she might go if she was to leave. When she looks back on her time in rehab the highlight for her was New Year's Eve. It was the closest that she came to being treated as an individual for some time.

MR: On New Year's Eve the orderly wheeled my bed out onto a balcony and it was a warm evening. I had a truly magnificent evening chatting and we had a few drinks and told jokes. I even had balloons tied to my bed. It was the best that I had felt for ages.

The golden rule in rehabilitation is that you can stay while you continue to improve. One day I was told that I would be discharged back to Tasmania. I was so frightened and alone; I had no idea what I was going to do. I was scared of the local hospital in Tasmania, but I had no choice. I had to go back. By the time I was back in Tasmania and in the hospital, I was quite sick again. I had to have an I.V. and a nasogastric tube and a catheter again. I was on a ward I had never been to, but it did not take long before they all seemed to know that the enigma had returned. The nurses were good to me though and were back to keeping a close eye on me.

I did not often see the doctors who cared for MR because I would visit in the evenings. However, on one occasion I did have an opportunity to talk with one of the doctors in the corridor. It was an awkward conversation because there was so much that I wanted to ask. He was on his way to see MR and he had her history with him. *'What do you think is going on?'* he asked me. I told him that MR had been admitted to this hospital some time ago with asthma. I wanted to state the obvious that she had asthma and now she was paralysed. I said that I was sure if he read the history somewhere in there he would locate when doctors began to believe that her condition was psychosomatic.

I told him that regardless of what her diagnosis was there seemed to be a rather large hole in the system that MR had fallen into. He looked confused and stood there rubbing his head. I also told him that I believed that whatever was written in her history was now very much part of her problem. He knew what I meant and he said *'It sure is a tricky one'*. He assured me that he was going to examine MR thoroughly. When I think back to this conversation he was telling me that as a doctor that was all he could do. He could examine her medically to see if there was some clue that might have eluded the attention of the many other doctors who had examined her before him. The only other thing that I said was *'It's awful isn't it'*. He nodded, sighed, and went to examine MR.

MR: The doctor actually examined me and commented on my poor condition. He seemed concerned. However, what he really thought, I will never know.

Not long after this MR began to feel healthier as the infections gradually cleared. Knowing that she would be facing being moved again she decided to ask if she could go to the rehabilitation unit in the hospital. The doctors agreed with her request and, after a much more positive experience on an acute ward than ever before, she was moved again.

11

HOME AT LAST

GIVING BACK THE BODY

MR returned to her quest to regain as much function as she could in her body and to continue where she had left off in Melbourne.

MR: I don't think the nurses liked touching me on the rehab ward and they just did not seem to wash me properly.

Because MR was in a rehabilitation ward the nurses attempted to give back some of the body care that had been done for her in the acute ward. However, MR had decided that to continue to survive she needed to be detached from her body as just a head again. The nurses tried to include her in their nursing care and to confront her with her body again—especially with what it could and could not do. Confronted with her body she could see how much she had deteriorated since she stopped having physiotherapy.

The nurses could well have perceived MR's behaviour as resistance on her part because on the rehabilitation ward they wanted to involve her with her care. MR had reserved the times that she was going to work on her body as those times that she spent with the physiotherapists. In fact, because the physiotherapists took her off the ward for exercise and treatment, the nurses were very disconnected from her progress. This fragmentation of care was confusing for MR especially since her physical times were only with the physiotherapists.

I have thought about this confusion often in relation to my own nursing practice because I had worked on a rehabilitation ward for some time at one stage in my nursing career. I remember caring for a man who was recovering after a car accident. When the doctors came to see him they asked *'Have you been for a walk today?'* *'Yes,'* he replied, *'twice with the physiotherapist'*. I was bewildered because we had spent the day walking together, but somehow they were not the important walks that he referred to.

I did not visit MR as much as I had previously while she was on the rehabilitation ward. When I did visit I had difficulty with her sense of hopelessness as nothing seemed to change except that she was even more ill. The big charts on the walls of MR's hospital room really depressed me as they displayed goals for her body, such as:

By Monday I will be able to wiggle all of my toes.

These charts were a stark reminder to all of us of what she could not do. I took some posters to put on her walls. I chose pictures of an astronaut walking in space, an eagle, a window with a view into a garden, and a wise-looking North American Indian. MR was amused at my choice of posters because she knew that they all represented movement. We talked about imagining movement and MR said that it was fun but that was all. I wanted to put up my posters so that other posters were not such a feature in her room.

MR: I think that I presented somewhat of a conundrum for the nurses because I wasn't a stroke or an amputee. They had looked after a woman with quadriplegia who was in the transition of going from a spinal unit to home. The nurses would say 'Well we did that for her, so it will work for you'. They made so many comparisons which started to irritate me because I was actually quite different with my lack of neck control, tiredness, and pain. More importantly I didn't want to be compared, because she would never get better and I believed that I would—or so I thought.

The term rehabilitation can mean many things in medicine and nursing. In general it is a broad term that refers to the provision of services to those who are disadvantaged. The medical usage of the term that is widely accepted tends to be the restoration of a person 'to the fullest physical, mental, social, vocational and economic usefulness of which they are capable' (Seymour 1989, p. 52). The problem with this Cartesian explanation of what rehabilitation might be is that it fails to incorporate an ethic of care 'which emphasises individuals and their rights, duties, and freedoms' (Wendall 1996, p. 139).

Susan Wendall (1996) has written from a feminist perspective a wonderfully insightful account of her experiences of living with a disability. After becoming ill with myalgic encephalomyelitis (ME) or chronic fatigue syndrome, she became aware and 'impressed by the knowledge people with disabilities have about living with bodily suffering and limitation and about how their cultures treat rejected aspects of bodily life' (Wendall 1996, p. 5). She argues that newly disabled people, such as MR, enter into a different world that they know little about because 'disabled people's experience is not integrated into the culture' (Wendall 1996, p. 65).

A STATE OF TURMOIL

MR: I remember a nurse who found it really difficult to cope with my mood swings. I was in a state of turmoil and I think she thought that I was deliberately obstructive. She would say to me 'Snap out of it' or 'Stop mucking around'. Once I got the flu and she said to me 'Oh no! Now we will have to blow your nose for you all of the time'. I quickly asked the doctor for an antihistamine to dry up my runny nose. The bonus was that it also made me very sleepy and thus provided me with some escape from everything.

The state of turmoil that MR refers to came about because she was confronted with her disability again, rather than being in hospital for a diagnosis and cure. Even though she had been paralysed for some time it had, mostly, been ignored until now. Her state of turmoil was added to by suggestions that she had the ability to control what was happening to her, such as that she could 'snap out of it'. The pressure for MR, as a patient worthy of rehabilitation, was that she must now improve. As I have implied throughout this book, MR had slowly lost more and more of her previous way of being and having a body. I can only ponder on why there had not been an intensive rehabilitation programme throughout her hospitalisation. The physiotherapy department was, after all, accessible from any other ward.

MR: I still had a Jason Recliner [chair] which was great, so that I could sit out of bed. However once I was washed and up I would be pushed over to the window and then I was on my own for hours. One day I graduated to a wheelchair and finally I could be moved around, and even off the ward. My mission became to get home and I really worked hard to achieve this. I hoped that more people would have come to see me at this stage, but visitors were still nearly non-existent. I did enjoy some regular phone calls from friends in Melbourne. However, I had plenty of distractions because there were many elderly people on the ward to talk to. I got on very well with them and they were not only encouraging but they were very supportive.

MAKING FRIENDS AGAIN

I remember that MR did begin to socialise with other people on the ward and this was certainly a change. She seemed to be reconnecting to the world outside of her bed and was rediscovering that social contact with people was still important to her. It was sad that when she most needed friends to visit her they, including myself, were nowhere to be found. Moore (1991, p. 143) states that 'One of the worst pains produced by the accident was the realisation that the support and friendship I needed during the hardest parts of my recovery were unavailable, unrecognised, unwanted or unembraced'. In the other people on the ward MR found friends and enjoyed the opportunity to share personal experiences of illness. This had not occurred much until now partly because she had been chronically ill, often living in an acute hospital bed.

MR: I even made a friend of a young guy with paraplegia. It was great to bounce off personal experiences with him and to share a joke but he really was very angry about what had happened to him.

MR may have been angry at times but, unlike her friend, she had no cause such as an accident or disease process to be angry with.

MR: Medically nothing changed much just the odd infection and asthma. Every now and then the nurses would take out my catheter to see if I could empty my bladder. I spent ages with taps running and water poured on my perineum—but it never worked. Once they thought I should have a ultrasound and you have to drink lots of water. There was a delay in proceedings and my bladder was enormous. As I sat in the corridor suddenly there was drip, drip as the urine by-passed my catheter and a puddle overflowed from my chair to the floor. I was so embarrassed but the staff were great about it.

For months I worked with the physios. There was everything from the tilt table to electrical stimulation. I did make some progress with my neck. Everyone reacted differently to my progress. Some were delighted at every small gain, I certainly was.

Wendall (1996, p. 98) discusses the pitfalls of seeking alternative therapeutic approaches for people with chronic illnesses. While she is specifically referring to Eastern or Chinese healing practices she makes the point that 'as long as the goal is to control the body, there is great potential in all healing practices for blaming the victims' (Wendall 1996, p. 98). There is a suggestion by MR that the nursing and medical staff believed that her slow improvement was because she did not really want to get better. MR speaks to this issue through her story.

MINIMAL PROGRESS

MR: Family meetings are a normal part of rehabilitation wherein all of the staff and the family meet to discuss progress. With no real family at hand, my meeting was just me and the staff. I was wheeled into a crowded room by a nurse. Only the doctor spoke and he said that there had been minimal progress and that it seemed that I may not make any further progress. I nearly fell out of my chair. I looked around the room with disbelief and everyone was gazing at their feet, obviously uncomfortable with what had been said. Surely I was going to get better. I was so upset that I really did not hear anything else that he said.

After the meeting I went to physio and I tried to put on a brave front but I started to weep. They all tried to comfort me but I felt as if the door had been closed on my life. I went back to my room and the nurses put me to bed and they closed the curtains around me because I was still crying. I desperately thought about what all of this might mean. There had to be something better than being a parasite on the health care system. I had to conjure up a survival system.

You have to make continual progress to stay on the rehab ward. I remember that day that they told me a nursing home was the only option for me.

MR was therefore blamed and punished for her minimal improvement because she had to leave the ward and go to a nursing home. Once again she has nowhere and no-one to turn to. MR believed that she had failed by not getting better and she calls herself a 'parasite on the health care system'. We can all identify with elderly people who say 'Don't put me into a nursing home', so it was reasonable to expect that a young woman would not want to live in a nursing home either.

MR: They insisted that I go and view this home. I was told that the home was for younger people with high levels of disability. I knew where it was, miles out of town and very isolated. Indeed it was very beautiful there, a really nice setting, right on a river surrounded by beautiful English trees. I sat there, by the river, and thought if only my wheelchair would run down the hill and tip me into the river so that I could drown.

I went inside and it was a huge place with single rooms. I happened to be there at lunch time and people were being fed. Some were badly disfigured, some were yelling out. The staff were very welcoming and seemed excited at the prospect of me living there. They seriously chatted to me about all of the afternoon activities that I could do. What a nightmare—I instantly hated the place. It wasn't the actual place I didn't like, it was the fear that my life was going to be reduced to this and afternoons of Bingo. I went back to the hospital and said categorically that no way could I possibly live there. I asked the doctor if I could live in my own home with carers. He didn't say no but explained the difficulties that I would face and expressed concern at the level of care that I would receive. In the end we agreed that if it didn't work out then I would go to the nursing home.

Once MR had exhibited symptoms similar to those with spinal injuries she probably should have had the same (albeit limited) opportunities that they do. At the initial stage of a spinal injury there is intensive injury management. Rehabilitation begins with an equally intensive physiotherapy and educational programme designed to teach the person how to live at home. All of the activities are designed for re-entry into the world and from the outset much of the person's day is taken up with intensive rehabilitation with planning for discharge interwoven throughout (Seymour 1989, p. 59). Even then after painstaking negotiation, Seymour (1989, p. 59) says that 'the return home can be a devastating experience'. MR had none of the opportunities that a person with a spinal injury would have had which is why the doctors had suggested a nursing home in the first place.

GOING HOME

MR: Then the race was on to get me home as the hospital would no longer provide a bed for me as a 'nursing home type patient'. Many of the nurses were concerned that my plan was doomed to fail and contended that I would not survive at home. The Occupational Therapist (OT) was wonderful and organised carers for me. I had a case manager and was given six months to prove that I could manage. I was not sure if I would be able to manage, but I was going home.

MR now had a 'case' manager. While I find the language problematic for obvious reasons, it was good that MR had someone to turn to for support and advice. When she went home her equipment seemed to fill up her cottage. She had a bed in a sunroom from where she could see her garden and her dog. MR's father had been doing some more renovations to her house for her return and he seemed overjoyed that she was home at last. MR lived with a friend whom she had worked with, so she was not always alone. Unfortunately this friendship later became strained and, as is the case for many people with disabilities, the friendship ended after a few months.

Wendall (1996, p. 129) draws our attention to the fact that people who are ill without a diagnosis often are not entitled to benefits and social programmes and many of them are abandoned by families and friends. Eventually MR was to lose most of her material possessions through her illness, such as her house and her car. Very quickly the money she did have got eaten up with all of her expenses. In the beginning though, her return home meant that friends did reappear to see her. I rather enjoyed visiting her at home although it did take me some time to get used to seeing her in a wheelchair in her old surroundings.

NEW ARMS AND LEGS

MR: My carers became my life-line, my new arms and legs. How I loved to be home and to be in control of how I was looked after. There was never enough care but what I did receive was good. With only four hours per day we were on a tight schedule but this became easier as time went by. There were minor disasters with equipment and tubing, but we managed and I never felt humiliated or a nuisance. Being at home was vastly superior to being in hospital. Another thing that was nice about being at home again was that visitors started to arrive again.

We are a society that offers very little by way of support for people with disabilities. The only thing that reminds us that people are living in the community with a disability are the larger car parking spots dotted around towns and cities. MR was able to visit the university but only because they had just put in a lift. However, when she organised to leave her home at other times, there were difficulties. Wheelchair access is a huge problem—it is very much a world for fit, active people.

One evening MR's house-mate called me to help pick her up after she had toppled out of the wheelchair. With great difficulty we got her back into the wheelchair. When MR had these accidents the full weight of her body would hit the floor, so she would sustain bruises and soreness for some time afterwards. There was not any carpet so she had fallen onto a hard surface. Somehow she would always add a little humour to these situations and we actually would have a laugh as we all got twisted and tangled helping her move. To manoeuvre people in hospitals there is equipment and attendants, but in MR's home nothing had been redesigned to make it more environmentally friendly for her. Most things were out of reach for MR because of high bench tops, knobs and handles, and the bathroom was a nightmare.

MR: I managed in my own home for some months and then to my surprise, my house-mate asked for a meeting between ourselves and my case manager. Apparently, she could not cope with living with me anymore because she found my carers and my new lifestyle too intrusive on her life. I guess that I was hurt that she had never spoken to me about the problems she was having. What hurt me more were the reasons she proffered, such as the top being left off the shampoo bottle or if the carer used one of her towels. It had all become too difficult and it seemed that my life was continuing its downward spiral.

I could not afford to pay the mortgage any longer as I was running out of money because work had stopped paying me and I was reliant on sickness benefits to pay a mortgage and all of the neverending bills that go with a chronic illness. I had no choice but to sell my home and move to a government supplied unit which was specially designed for a wheelchair.

Sadly MR and her house-mate did not discuss any of the issues that became real problems for both of them. It was not hard to understand many of the problems that faced them both as soon as MR was living at home again. I did talk with her house-mate and, obviously, tops left off shampoo bottles and towels, were not the real issues. Sadly, neither of them had the opportunity to talk about the 'real' problems then or later, and what was a friendship came to an end. Lately I have thought about how important it was to address the issues at the time because MR is still angry about the meeting she refers to that precipitated her friendship ending and leaving her home. I believe that MR and her house-mate's unresolved problems reflect the broader issue of the inadequate support available in the community for the 'carers' (families and friends) of people who are chronically ill living at home.

MR moved into her new unit and it all went well for a time until MR had bouts of infections that meant she was in and out of hospital again. She still had a catheter and, because of swallowing difficulties, was having enteral feeding.

SURRENDERING TO THE 'FIGHT'

MR: By January 1995 I felt that my life was falling apart. I had been sick almost constantly with various infections and asthma. I would get over one problem and then another one would hit me. A severe bout of pleurisy and pneumonia made breathing extremely difficult and I had spent time gurgling in hospital. My friend was over from Melbourne and I couldn't even enjoy her visit. Also my eyesight seemed to be deteriorating and I even had trouble watching the mindless television. I was exhausted and fed up with how hard my existence was. Rumours were around that I may lose my carers. Apparently they were only allowed to look after people who were medically stable. I often refused to go to hospital and

I think that it was unfair of me to place this burden on the carers, but I was determined that if I was going to die it was not going to be alone in a hospital where I had experienced so much pain. There were no good days any more and no quality to my life that motivated me to cling to my life. No one could promise me things could be better and I couldn't promise anything better for myself.

On 18 January I decided to surrender the fight. It was time to die. I met with my case manager who I really respected and enjoyed talking to. She said to me 'It's not looking good; what do you want to do?' I told her that I wanted to die and she said 'I know'. I cried then. It was so cathartic to talk about what I was feeling.

MR describes her illness as a war that she has fought for some time. Sontag (1990) discusses the military metaphors that surround cancer but she argues that society has also declared war on cancer. MR's battle was entirely personal and I had never heard her use the metaphors of war before.

MR: I decided that I would withdraw all of my treatment on 25 January including my enteral feeds.

At first I had an outpouring of sadness and grief but then I actually felt peaceful for the first time in two years. My friend Lesley came to see me and we both cried when I told her, and the case manager said that she would talk with my doctor and my father. Lesley spent a great deal of time with me going through my things for me. Then my best friend Sally rang and she was indignant about my decision. I had to reassure and comfort her. Sally decided to fly over and come and see me.

Word of my decision spread very quickly and in no time everyone knew. I was lectured on the errors of my ways. People would tell me that I was young with so much to give. I think in the Western world people are hung up on the quantity of life, not the quality, and people are afraid of death. This was not an impulsive decision but one that had evolved over a long period of time. This was not existence but subsistence. Death held no fear for me, but I was petrified as to how I would die. I did not want to die in a hospital alone and I did not want to die being unable to breathe.

SICK TODAY, WELL TOMORROW

This is the beginning of MR telling the narrative that has come to dominate her story of illness. She came to this narrative through suffering and pain. As MR began to tell this story the people around her began to pressure her to tell what Frank (1995, p. 77) calls restitution narratives. According to Frank (1995, p. 77) this narrative has 'the basic storyline: "Yesterday I was healthy, today I'm sick, but tomorrow I'll be healthy again"'. The assumption is that anyone who is sick wants to be healthy again and ill people are expected to tell this story rather than 'that they have had enough and they want to die'.

MR: My next hurdle was my doctor, who was shocked but understanding. He was concerned that I had become depressed and he suggested antidepressants. I told him that I was depressed but only commensurate with the reality of my existence. My doctor insisted that I see a psychiatrist and I was happy to do that so that it would help him. He also said that he would have to seek legal advice. I could understand all of this and he was very supportive even though his aim was to get me to reconsider. The doctor talked about nursing homes again but I explained I had just fought for two years to keep out of one. I do know that he understood and he said he knew many people who would want to do the same thing if they were in my position.

Frank (1995, p. 83) tells us that the restitution narrative is 'the culturally preferred narrative'. However for some people 'eventually the reality and responsibility of mortality, and its mystery, have to be faced' (Frank 1995, p. 84). The doctor offering antidepressants offers the medical restitution narrative, but we hear MR resist this story for her own.

MR: The community nurses also understood my decision. Not one of them changed in the way that I was cared for as a result of my decision. My carers were given the choice as to whether they would stay or leave—they all stayed. I received flowers, letters, and phone calls from friends and family. One friend, Patrick, sent me a beautiful tape which contained readings from *The Tibetan Book of Living and Dying*. Everything was falling into place.

Many people, including the nurses, allowed MR to tell her story and did not pressure her to tell the story of being well.

MR: Some friends had discussions and offered to take it in turns to be with me. I can never thank them for all they did for me at this time. I made my own funeral arrangements—the cheapest that I could get was $1800. I organised a will and saw the psychiatrist. We had a reasonable conversation about why I wanted to die. She told me it was OK to change my mind.

Everything was going to plan except that the doctor started to waver slightly and Denise started to interfere. She seemed concerned that there were nursing students there. We argued about it.

THE ANGRY FRIEND

I was angry. Not sad that MR might die; not understanding that she wanted to die; just angry. I thought that the whole scene reminded me of a slow motion, badly scripted film that I wanted to turn off. I intellectualised and theorised what everyone was doing and that did not help. I decided that I did not want to be part of it. I thought that the way that she would die, through no hydration and nutrition, was not going to be a good death. MR told me that I had interfered because I wanted to discuss some of the issues that concerned me with the two nursing students who were also her friends. I think I was imagining an inquest after she was dead and being asked '*As a registered nurse and a lecturer in nursing, did you ever have a conversation with the two students involved in this case?*'

The other issue for me was that I did not believe that MR wanted to die. When we argued I was glad she was angry with me and I did not regret that conversation. I felt that she ran rings around me with her arguments and I remember feeling scared of her. I had seen her angry when she had been well, but not since. I wondered if MR was testing out how much she meant to people. I was confused because I have been with and supported many people when they have died. I have been with people when life support has been turned off, when medications have been altered that have contributed to an earlier, but inevitable, death. However this confronted me with an ethical and moral dilemma that I was not familiar with.

If MR had told me she was going to press a button to receive a lethal injection maybe I would have been less confronted, but I don't really know that either. Although in general people believe that with 'drugs' death can be comfortable and good, that has not always been my experience of death as a nurse. Everybody was so quiet and accepting—except me. There were hushed tones around the bed. I kept thinking *'Where were you all over the last few years; why are you all here now?'* Yes, I was very angry and not just with MR. I did not say to her *'You can be better,'* or *'There will be a better life,'* or even *'You have so much to give'*—because I did not believe that either.

MR: On 25 January I had my pump turned off. I would never have to hear that irritating drone again. There was one last thing that I wanted to do, I wanted to fly in a small plane over Cradle Mountain. My friends arranged it and propped up with pillows we went skyward, the clouds cleared as if on cue. The view was fantastic. I was delighted to see patches of snow. I closed my eyes to see if I could imagine being dead, I was ready to die.

After the flight MR went home to die. One evening she was at home in her bed, alone for a moment until the next carer arrived, when her doctor visited. She could not let him in so he climbed through the window. He had a lengthy talk with MR and told her that life could be different and that he could organise another hospital in Melbourne that would take her. The doctor spoke the medical restitution narrative to forestall MR's story. I know this doctor and MR had him as her GP because she had great respect for him. I can only imagine how desperate he must have felt, because MR said he pleaded with her to reconsider.

RESUMING THE FIGHT

After painstaking deliberation MR heard the doctor's plea and decided to live in Melbourne again. I know that many times since she has regretted the decision she made then and is angry that the future the doctor described to her never eventuated. MR was angry with the doctor because she still believed that medicine had the answers. The doctor was able to dominate her story with the more culturally-preferred story. A doctor and a nurse (me) had been MR's only resistance. So, what of choice and a person's rights? I do not discuss the ethical and moral issues here, but MR has pursued this in detail and has entered into the euthanasia debate on national television and in the newsprint media.

On the *Today Show* Steve Liebmann captured the culturally preferred restitution story beautifully. From what I can remember he said that to look at MR she seemed young, articulate and intelligent so therefore she had so much to give. And there was the guilt trip thrown in as well when he compared her to those who will die but want to live. He remarked that there are so many people worse off than her. In fact I remember how confronted he seemed by MR's articulate intelligence and because she did not tell her story of pain and suffering he made inaccurate assumptions about her life.

MR: Some people ask me how I can think about dying when I am so intelligent and articulate. You cannot compare my situation with others. It is not up to people to devise a scale of suffering; it is not reality and is extremely ignorant. That is certainly what the *Today Show* said to me.

MR had struggled throughout her illness with people not believing she was really ill and, ironically, now I did not believe that she really wanted to die. Maybe it was because I expected to hear the restitution narrative, that Frank (1995) describes, that I was so uncomfortable. Maybe because I had been listening to her story so closely, I had decided how the story might continue for me rather than her. Needless to say, both MR and I have changed a great deal since then in our understandings of life and death.

MR prepared to go and live in Melbourne again.

12

BEING AN INSTITUTIONALISED BODY

MISSING MY LEGS

MR went to Melbourne again and has lived there ever since. She went to the hospital that the doctor had suggested and a less intensive rehabilitation programme was commenced. I visited MR in the hospital in Melbourne. As I made my way through the wards to see her I was encouraged by the warm environment. It seemed as if there had been major renovations as evidenced by fresh paint, new curtains and comfortable-looking beds. But, as I found my way to MR, the environment deteriorated markedly. It reminded me of the older sections of the hospital where I had trained in as a nurse and familiar sights and sounds greeted me.

When I opened the door to the ward I set off the alarm and a loud sound announced my arrival—everyone looked my way. The first person that I saw was a scantily clad man in a wheelchair going for a bath. There was no privacy for anyone in architecture such as this. I scanned the rooms of beds for MR—people were calling out and wailing. I knew when I had found MR's room because I recognised her wheelchair and her belongings which seemed to spill out of her small designated area. The screens were closed and I could see the shape of the nurse as she moved around the bed half draped in the curtain. They were preparing for my visit.

The nurse gave me instructions on how to leave without setting off the alarm and then she said that I could go in. MR was lying on her side and she looked pale but better than the last time that I had seen her. Her hair had grown and it was a beautiful golden colour. She had no catheter and no feeding pump but I could see that she could not move. We had a glass of champagne. MR said that it was on her medication chart, we giggled and I hid the bottle. I held her glass and the straw—it was good to see her. She had a view from her bed into a courtyard with trees and a water fountain. As we talked she would often stare outside. I read to her what I had written. She listened intently as I read to her, and, as was our custom, she would interrupt to discuss what I was saying. I recorded her responses to what I had written on that day.

MR: When Denise reads this to me or I read it myself it is still the right story. Even now, that's how it was; that's how I felt. It all seems like a bad dream. It's been so long—I've been so sick. I listen to my story and I think, why wasn't I more pro-active? But I was just not well enough. I remember a full life and suddenly it was taken away from me. I have felt loss and grief.

I really miss my legs. I remember the sound of my feet on the bridge where I lived; the sound of my feet walking. The wind in my hair.

I should have looked after myself better—not worked so hard. I still know that something happened to me at that time. I couldn't control it, and I can't explain it . . .

If I had been in another hospital maybe action would have been taken earlier to stop me deteriorating so dramatically; maybe they would have discovered what was going on. I think that I was left too long. Maybe I would have had more of a chance if the medical profession weren't so narrow-minded. Doctors are fallible and they may not always have the patient's best interests at heart. It puzzles me that doctors don't have the same curiosity that scientists have to find answers. They test for things that already exist. If they can't find the answer in the 'body', why do they think it's in the 'head'? And then why do they not consider that the 'head' is a valid thing to treat?

Pain is a big part of my life now, and of course it cannot be explained. I truly, deeply believe something happened to me, but at times now I question and doubt my own intuitive feelings about my body. I do know my body and I like to think I have always been honest about it to the doctors. I don't think they heard me.

I have been frustrated, angry, sad; and I grieve and I cry. I mainly cry for the other people I meet who are ill. People tend not to leave here and I have witnessed some tragedies.

I am not a better person for being ill. I wasn't a bad person before I was ill, and I am still basically the same person. I am becoming more aware of my body. My pain reminds me of my body. People don't ask me what is wrong with me any more; they assume I have been in a car accident. But, if they ask, I say, 'I've got a rare neurological disease'.

In some ways I'm not comfortable reading my story, but that's how I felt. It has captured lots of things; lots of things that happened. Yes, I like it . . . it's good. It says a lot.

I am beginning to feel a sense of time passing. I am worried that I am missing what was going to have been the prime of my life. I think about having children, but I know that I will never have any of my own. I still grieve for that loss especially now that I see my friends having their families. I *am* going to look after myself. I am absolutely determined. I am different from most who are ill; it is very different having an illness that cannot be attributed to anything. It makes the whole experience different. And harder.

A diagnosis was not relevant at first, but as I became chronically ill it became more of an issue. There was the reality of a catheter, a feeding tube, of not being able to walk, and of no explanations.

There is never a time when I don't want to get better. I have so much to gain from getting better—what sort of existence is this? Rules, regulations . . . I wanted to live. I wanted to have children.

Initially I expected to get better; now I know I will not get better. No-one ever intimates that I might not want to get better. I think that my friends now accept that this is how I am going to be. I am not always happy.

The thing that stands out the most for me from telling this story is I would say the focus of your mind becomes your body in an institution. It is part of being institutionalised.

Something happened to me. I will never accept it was or is psychosomatic . . . what does that mean anyway? I think I was abandoned. Yes . . . they abandoned me!

THE NURSING HOME

MR was eventually to lose her struggle to stay out of a nursing home. There did not seem to be any other alternatives—she had tried them all. When a bed became available MR left the hospital for a nursing home.

MR: I think it is important not to dwell on how I am now because I know that I won't get better—I've tried. I have put my best effort into that and now I haven't got the strength. My life force is not so strong—it's wavering and it gets less. Yes I do want to get better and I have been very angry about being so ill. I have got something I would call faith in myself; you know I am comfortable with myself. I like to think of the time/space continuum that I am passing through—sort of a Buddhist thing. I think I've been close to death quite often and it's not a tangible thing—it's just something you know. It's like a flickering candle burning out. I might stop breathing maybe, but I am ready to die.

When I think of how I was, I try to understand my former existence. I get lost and I think 'Have I always been like this?' My existence is a reflection of my body and illness. Does anyone understand how important my life has been to me? My world is small but it is only bounded by mind and my mind is huge. I tap into the world through friends and cyberspace. Maybe I should ask my friends, 'What do you see me as?' Maybe they see me as just a head. Sometimes I don't think of anything really—I just am, I am alive.

When you say that I am a young woman with quadriplegia and multiple medical problems it makes me sound pathetic. Someone not part of society, put away in a nursing home—incarcerated. I am not pathetic although I may be an enigma.

My thoughts have turned to dying and to my own mortality again. I began to think about the losses which have accompanied my illness and what would never be. Pain was also and still is a constant factor in my life. It's the kind of pain which permeates my every waking moment and disturbs my sleep. Pain and tiredness dominate my life. The place where I have the least pain is when I am lying in bed. Any movement causes me pain and most of the nurses know how to touch me without causing too much pain. I don't get out into the chair very often because of the pain.

Personal pain is very difficult to explain to others, especially to doctors. It has been very difficult to get the doctors to deal with my pain or even acknowledge that it exists. I understand that you can't see the pain but I'm not the sort of person that rolls around the bed moaning. I prefer to lie quietly to deal with my pain. An assumption is often made by people that palliative care and pain management is effective now and can help everyone. The people who say this are not in pain and have no idea of the reality of the situation.

Let me just tell you about loss. I have lost many friends. Some believe that I have brought all of this on myself. I did have a house-mate who initially stuck by me when I returned home but the reality of my condition was just too harsh for her. Watching your friendship deteriorate is difficult. Sometimes I had only spasmodic contact with Denise; she would phone me up out of the blue. Once she phoned me on New Year's Eve. I told her I was having a truly magnificent time.

When I was in hospital in Tasmania I saw very little of my local friends. I think my undiagnosed illness affected their attitude towards me. Launceston is a small town and it was rife with gossip about me bringing it all on to myself. When I lost my job no one said thank you for my contribution at work; it was as if I never existed. They just put all of my things in a box at the back of a room. To see the life that you thrived on crammed into a box was the most devastating personal event of my illness. I have never forgotten it or the superficiality of people towards me.

So what is it I see for my future, in terms of dying. Well, it's difficult to have control over your life when you are chronically ill. I do not want to die in a hospital. We are so caught up on keeping people alive as long as possible. I want the right to have the choice to die so I am fighting for the choice to die by euthanasia. That choice should be there if life becomes unbearable because of chronic or terminal illness.

I don't know how much time in this life I have left, but time is precious and I will not waste it. The first 26 years of my life were fantastic. Now I am going to prepare my friends for my death so that they may understand and feel happy that my many sufferings are finally over when I do die. I am ready for the final chapter of my life.

REFLECTIONS

Denise Fassett

As this book draws to an end I struggle with what to say about a woman who has endured so much. I find I am left with all of the questions I started with and so many more, but I am left with some different understandings of MR, of myself, of nursing, and of being ill. Being with MR when she made that abrupt transition into the 'kingdom of the sick' will always haunt me. I doubt we will ever know what happened to her as she took her last steps before she became so ill. I remember the warm afternoon, the shimmer of light on the river, and the stillness of the bush that echoed our talking and laughter. And I remember the look on MR's face as she went through the doors into ICU. These images are always together for me.

Even now, when I read the story that MR has told and I have written, I am surprised. This is not the story I expected MR to tell. I did not ever expect MR to objectify her body to the extent that she does. If MR had been given a diagnosis her story would surely have been a different version of being a medicalised body. I doubt I would be any more comfortable with that story but, given MR's beliefs about medical boxes and medical salvation, I'm sure she would be.

I had believed that I would have been able to write that, despite Cartesian constructions of the body in health care, MR did not experience being a Cartesian body—but she did and may have always, but never to the extent of being just a head. MR was forced into being Cartesian about herself if she was to remain legitimate as a patient without a diagnosis. The consequences of this were that her story helped shape a reality of MR always being other to her self. The reductionist mind–body split was reinforced for MR by everyone, including me—until she was cast aside to life in an institution.

Cartesian understandings of the body are a discursive trap for us all and these understandings are embedded in our culture through our language and thus our stories. MR's story reveals, if only partially, how the narrative structure of stories are shaped within the totalising narratives of modernity. The mechanistic constructions of the body shape the way we nurse and the ways in which people experience illness. As MR became ill it was evident that she was comfortable being a Cartesian body. Later, however, she may have felt that science had turned its back on her. I certainly do.

Through MR's illness narrative she identified her 'self' through the medical, scientific discourse as consciousness and an object body. She described herself as just a head and argues that she gave up her body to be cared for. She also alluded to the ambiguity of such a statement by saying that some nurses did not look after just a body, they cared for her and were described by MR as part of her embodiment. This analysis touches only briefly on the complexity of theorising the body, the problem of the body, and the interactions that nurses have with people in their day-to-day work. When it was suggested that her illness was not real, many nurses and all of the doctors struggled with what to do with MR's body. It would seem that many, not knowing what to do, abandoned her. There were only a few nurses who continued to care for her sensitively despite her lack of a diagnosis.

The incompatibility of the experience of being ill and of receiving therapeutic health care is inscribed on the bodies of those who become ill. Nurses know this. They live with this tension every day through the stories and experiences of those they care for, but they seldom explore what it might mean. This narrative may help in raising some of these issues by illuminating the tensions that exist between embodiment and science. Other tensions that are evident in this book, such as how to speak for the self and others and how to theorise the body without losing 'real bodies', remain challenges for future scholarship.

BEING A BETTER PERSON

We are often led to believe that people who have extreme changes in their lives through illness, somehow learn from them and become better people than they were before. MR disagrees as she says she was not a bad person before she was ill. Perhaps it is as Sacks proposes that being ill forces us to 'scrutinise the deepest, darkest, and most fearful part of ourselves'.

> Force of habit and resistance to change—so great in all realms of thought—reaches its maximum in medicine, in the study of our most complex sufferings and disorders of being; for we are here compelled to scrutinise the deepest, darkest, and most fearful parts of ourselves, the parts we all strive to deny or not to see. The thoughts which are most difficult to grasp or express are those which touch on this forbidden region and re-awaken in us our strongest denials and our most profound intuitions. (Sacks 1991, p. xix)

These days MR's thin, frail body is turned every two hours by the nurses and years of immobility are written upon her body. Her voice-activated computer is her only means of daily communication with the outside world unless she ventures out in her electric wheelchair. Despite all of this though she is still always ready to talk, her quick wit ever present. And, she was and is always the scientist ever vigilant in her belief that the real diagnosis has been overlooked.

Since that eventful walk, MR has spent most of her time in and out of health care institutions slowly losing more and more of her previous ways of having and being a body. Her experiences of being a patient continue as she lies in a nursing home in Melbourne, Australia. MR's world has been totally transformed. Although her condition changes she is now living with all of the potential infections and complications of having and being a body which no longer moves.

As much as I have enjoyed writing this book there have been many times that it has seemed daunting because I have listened and been part of MR's story over a number of years. Selecting those aspects of her story that appear in this book was difficult. Although I have not included any of MR's experiences of living in the nursing home directly, some of those experiences are interwoven in all of the chapters because of the retrospective way that the story is told.

Reflections

I have visited MR a few times in the nursing home. Her room is dominated by her bed and computer, but it is a friendly room. I wondered what it was like to have a computer as a life-line—what did life in cyberspace have to offer? The last time I visited, MR sent me to the supermarket to buy lunch. We had a bottle of champagne, hommos, a little taste of smoked salmon and soft bread. I really enjoyed having lunch with her. What struck me about my visit though was the fact that I could leave and she could not. I got on the train after my visit and felt really troubled, perhaps even guilty, leaving her in the nursing home.

Writing these last words is very freeing for me because I know that I need to go back to being MR's friend again, rather than being the co-researcher or co-author. As I have said in the book, stories change in every telling and this one is no exception. I have shuffled some places and events around so that specific people will not be able to identify themselves, but inevitably I believe that everyone who reads this will see themselves in these stories.

It took me a long time before I finally walked the Duck Reach track again but I was glad that I did. It was just as beautiful and it gave me the opportunity to think about MR. I have often wondered how I would have coped if I had become ill as she has. I think that I would have searched for a diagnosis but I'm unsure as to how I would have ever managed to survive the ordeal. I have learned a great deal through MR's experiences that I believe have been important and significant in my life as a woman and as a nurse. I am fearful of illness. I know that I have, indeed we all have, what Sontag describes as a passport for wellness that could expire at any time. I like to believe that understandings of illness and disability will be incorporated gradually into our general cultural understandings of what it means to be a person.

There are no answers or conclusions from the telling of this story but there are most certainly many questions and challenges for everyone as we approach the next century. I believe that medicine will change as a discipline in response to people's experiences, but maybe not in my lifetime. Nurses, and other health professionals, however, can respond to the call from ill people and they can do it now. I believe we have much to learn from people who are ill and that ill people need those who are well to assist them to navigate their lives while they might have momentarily lost their way.

Just a Head

I am sad when I read MR's story—it is the pain in her story that reaches out and touches me. MR tells me she wants to die but while she is alive she will live. I understand that now.

REFERENCES

Belenky, M.F., Clinchy, B.M., Goldberger, N.R., and Tarule, J.M. 1986, *Women's Ways Of Knowing: The Development of Self, Voice, and Mind*, Basic Books, New York

Benhabib, S. 1992, *Situating the Self, Community and Postmodernism in Contemporary Ethics*, Polity Press, Oxford

Benner, P. and Wrubel, J. 1989, *The Primacy of Caring: Stress and Coping in Health and Illness*, Addison-Wesley, Menlo Park

Benner, P. 1984, *From Novice to Expert: Excellence and Power in Clinical Nursing Practice*, Addison-Wesley, Menlo Park

———1991, 'The role of experience, narrative, and community in skilled ethical comportment', *Advances In Nursing Science*, vol. 14, no. 2, pp. 1–21

Benoist, J. and Cathebras, P. 1993, 'The body: from immateriality to another', *Social Science and Medicine*, vol. 7, no. 36, pp. 857–65

Bernstein, R. 1983, *Beyond Objectivism and Relativism: Science, Hermeneutics, and Praxis*, University of Pennsylvania Press, Philadelphia

Bordo, S.R. 1989, 'The body and the reproduction of femininity: A feminist appropriation of Foucault', in A.M. Jaggar and S.R. Bordo (eds), *Gender/Body/Knowledge: Feminist Reconstructions of Being and Knowing*, Rutgers University Press, New Brunswick

———1990, 'Reading the slender body', in M. Jacobus, E.F. Keller and S. Shuttleworth (eds), *Body/Politics: Women and the Discourses of Science*, Routledge, New York

———1993, 'Feminism, Foucault and the politics of the body', in

C. Ramazanoglu (ed.), *Up Against Foucault: Exploration of some Tensions between Foucault and Feminism*, Routledge, London

Butler, J. 1993, *Bodies That Matter: On the Discursive Limits of Sex*, Routledge, London

Campbell, J. and Bunting, S. 1991, 'Voices and Paradigms: Perspectives on critical and feminist theory in nursing', *Advances in Nursing Science*, vol. 13, no. 3, pp. 1–15

Capra, F. 1982, *The Turning Point, Science, Society and the Rising Culture*, Flamingo, Harper Collins Book Manufacturing, Glasgow

Chalmers, A.F. 1976, *What is this Thing called Science*, University of Queensland Press, Queensland

Charlesworth M. 1982, *Science, Non-Science and Pseudo-Science*, Deakin University Press, Victoria

Cixous, H. 1981, 'Castration or Decapitation?', *Signs: Journal of Women in Culture and Society*, vol. 7, no. 1, pp. 41–55

Cohler, B. J. 1982, 'Personal narrative and life course', *Life-Span Development and Behaviour*, no. 4, pp. 205–41

Colliere, M.F. 1986, 'Invisible care and invisible women as health care-providers', *International Nursing Review*, vol. 7, no. 39, pp. 95–112

Connors, D. 1985, 'Women's "sickness": a case of secondary gains or primary losses', *Advances in Nursing Science*, vol. 7, no. 2, pp. 1–17

Cranny-Francis, A. 1995, *The Body in the Text*, Melbourne University, Carlton, Victoria

Dallery, A. B. 1989, 'The politics of writing (the) body: Ecriture feminine', in A.M. Jaggar and S.R. Bordo (eds), *Gender/Body/Knowledge: Feminist Reconstructions of Being and Knowing*, Rutgers University Press, New Brunswick

De Concini, B. 1990, *Narrative Remembering*, University of America Press, Lanham

Dickson, G. 1990, 'A feminist poststructuralist analysis of the knowledge of menopause', *Advances In Nursing Science*, vol. 12, no. 3, pp. 15–31

Diprose, R. 1991, 'A "genethics" that makes sense', in R. Diprose and R. Ferrell (eds), *Cartographies: Poststructuralism and the Mapping of Bodies and Spaces*, Allen & Unwin, St Leonards, Australia

——1994, *The Bodies of Women: Ethics, Embodiment and Sexual Difference*, Routledge, London

Dreyfus, H.L. 1976, Forward to the California edn, in Foucault, M. 1976, *Mental Illness and Psychology*, University of California Press, Los Angeles

Foucault, M. 1965, *Madness and Civilization, a History of Insanity in the Age of Reason*, Tavistock Publications, London

——1973, *The Birth of the Clinic: An Archaeology of Medical Perception*, trans. A.M. Sheridan Smith, Tavistock Publications, London

——1976a, *Mental Illness and Psychology*, University of California Press, Los Angeles, London

References

———1976b, *The History of Sexuality: Volume 3, The Care of the Self*, trans., R. Hurley, Penguin Books, London
———1977, *Discipline and Punish, the Birth of the Prison*, trans. A. Sheridan, Penguin Books, London
———1980, *Power/Knowledge: Selected Interviews and other Writings*, ed. G. Gordon, Pantheon, New York
———1988, 'Technologies of the self', in L.H. Martin, H. Gutman and P.H. Hutton (eds), *Technologies of the self: A Seminar with Michel Foucault*, The University of Massachusetts Press, Amherst
Frank, A.W. 1990, 'Bringing bodies back in: A decade review', *Theory, Culture and Society*, vol. 7, pp. 131–62
———1991, *At the Will of the Body: Reflections on Illness*, Houghton Mifflin Company, Boston
———1995, *The Wounded Story Teller. Body Illness and Ethics*, The University of Chicago Press, Chicago and London
Gadow, S. 1982, 'Body and self: A dialectic', in V. Kestenbaum (ed.), *The Humanity of the Ill: Phenomenological Perspectives*, University of Tennessee Press, Knoxville
Game, A. and Pringle, R. 1983, *Gender at Work*, George Allen and Unwin, Sydney
Garmanikow, E. 1978, 'Sexual Division of Labour: in the case of nursing', in Kuhn, A. and Wolpe, A.M. (eds), *Feminism and Materialism*, Routledge and Kegan Paul, London
Gatens, M. 1988, 'Towards a feminist theory of the body', in B. Caine, E. Grosz and M. de Lepervanche (eds), *Crossing Boundaries: Feminisms and the Critique of Knowledges*, Allen & Unwin, Sydney
———1996, *Imaginary Bodies: Ethics, Power and Corporeality*, Routledge, London
Gluck, S.B. and Patai D. 1991, *Women's Words: The Feminist Practice of Oral History*, Routledge, London
Grosz, E. and de Lepervanche, M. 1988, 'Feminism and Science', in B. Caine, E. Grosz, and M. de Lepervanche (eds), *Crossing Boundaries: Feminisms and the Critique of Knowledges*, Allen & Unwin, Sydney
Grosz, E. 1992, *Sexual Subversions: Three French Feminists*, Allen & Unwin, Sydney
———1994, *Volatile Bodies: Toward a Corporeal Feminism*, Allen & Unwin, Sydney
Harth, E, 1992, *Cartesian Women: Versions and Subversions of Rational Discourse in the Old Régime*, Cornell University Press, New York
Hays, J. C. 1989, 'Voices in the record', *Image: Journal of Nursing Scholarship*, vol. 21, no. 4, pp. 200–4
Holmes, C. A. 1994, 'Nursing's construction of the body', in B. Turner, L. Eckerman, D. Colquhoun and P. Crotty (eds), *Embodiment, Annual Review of Health Social Sciences, Volume Four*, Centre for the Body and Society, Deakin University, Geelong

hooks, bell 1990, *Yearning, race, gender, and cultural politics*, South End Press, Boston

Horsfall, J. 1997, 'Some consequences of the psychiatric dis-integration of the body, mind and soul', in Lawler J. (ed.), *The Body in nursing*, Churchill Livingstone, Melbourne

Hubbard, R. 1990, *The Politics Of Women's Biology*, Rutgers University Press, New Brunswick

Kelber, W.H. 1990, 'Narrative as interpretation and interpretation of narrative: Hermeneutical reflections on the Gospels', in T. Maranhao (ed.), *The Interpretation of Dialogue*, The University of Chicago Press, Chicago

Keller, E.F. 1985, *Reflections on Gender and Science*, Yale University Press, New Haven

——1989. 'The Gender/Science System: or, Is Sex to Gender as nature Is to Science?', in Tuana, N. (ed.), *Feminism and Science*, Indiana University Press, Indiana, USA

Kleinman, A. 1988, *The Illness Narratives*, Basic Books, New York

Kramarae, C. and Spender, D. 1992, in C. Kramarae and D. Spender (eds), *The Knowledge Explosion: Generations Of Feminist Scholarship*, Teachers College Press, New York

Kuhn, T.S. 1970, *The Structure of Scientific Revolutions*, The University of Chicago Press, Chicago

Laqueur, T. 1990, *Making Sex: Body And Gender From The Greeks to Freud*, Harvard University Press, Cambridge

Lather, P. 1991, *Getting Smart: Feminist Research and Pedagogy With/In the PostModern*, Routledge, London

——1993, 'The politics and ethics of feminist research: researching the lives of women with HIV/AIDS', Draft paper for the *Ethnography and Education Research Forum*, Philadelphia (unpub.)

Lawler, J. 1991, *Behind the Screens: Nursing Somology, and the Problem of the Body*, Churchill Livingstone, Melbourne

——1997, 'Knowing the body and embodiment; methodologies, discourses and nursing', in Lawler (ed.), *The Body in nursing*, Churchill Livingstone, Melbourne

Leder, D. 1984, 'Medicine and paradigms of embodiment', *Journal of Medical Philosophy*, vol. 9, pp. 29–43

Lumby, J. 1992, 'Making meaning from a woman's experience of illness: The emergence of a feminist method for nursing', unpublished doctoral dissertation, Deakin University, Geelong

Lupton, L. 1996, *Food, the Body and the Self*, Sage Publications, London

Lyotard, J.F. 1984, *The Postmodern Condition: A Report on Knowledge*, trans. G. Bennington and B. Massouri, University of Minnesota Press, Minneapolis

MacSween, M. 1993, *Anorexic Bodies. A feminist and sociological perspective on anorexia nervosa*, Routledge, London

REFERENCES

Madjar, I. 1997 'The body in health, illness and pain', in Lawler, J. (ed.), *The Body in Nursing*, Churchill Livingstone, Melbourne

Magee, B. 1987, *The Great Philosophers*, BBC Books, London

Martin, E. 1987, *The Woman in the Body, A Cultural Analysis of Reproduction*, Open University Press, Milton Keynes, UK

Matthews, A. 1986, 'Patient-centred handovers', *Nursing Times*, vol. 82, no. 24, pp. 47–8

McInerney, F. 1992, 'Provision of food and fluids in terminal care: a sociological analysis', *Social Science and Medicine*, vol. 34, no. 11, pp. 1271–6

McLaren, P. 1988, 'Schooling the postmodern body: Critical pedagogy and the politics of enfleshment', *Journal of Education*, vol. 170, no. 3, pp. 53–83

McMahon, B. 1994, 'The functions of space', *Journal of Advanced Nursing*, vol. 19, pp. 362–6

Minh-Ha T.T. 1991, *When The Moon Waxes Red: Representation, Gender And Cultural Politics*, Routledge, New York

Monahan, M. 1988, 'Change of shift report: a time for communication with patients', *Nursing Management*, vol. 19, no. 2, p. 80

Moore, T. 1991, *Cry of the Damaged Man, a Personal Journey of Recovery*, Picador, Australia

Namenwirth, M. 1986, 'Science seen through a feminist prism', in R. Bleier (ed.), *Feminist Approaches To Science*, Pergamon Press Inc., New York

Nancy, J. 1994, 'Corpus', in Flower MacCannell, J. and Zacharin L. (eds), *Thinking Bodies*, Stanford University Press, Stanford, California

Parker, J.M. 1988, 'Theoretical perspectives in nursing: from microphysics to hermeneutics', paper presented at the Third Nursing Research Forum, *Shaping Nursing Theory and Practice: The Australian Context*, March, Melbourne, Australia

——1991a, 'Being and nature: An interpretation of person and environment', in G. Gray and R. Pratt (eds), *Towards a Discipline of Nursing*, Churchill Livingstone, Melbourne

——1991b, 'Bodies and boundaries in nursing: A postmodern and feminist analysis', paper given at the National Nursing Conference, *Science, Reflectivity and Nursing Care: exploring the Dialectic*, December 5 and 6, Melbourne, Australia

——1997, 'The body as text and the body as living flesh: metaphors of the body and nursing in postmodernity', in Lawler, J. (ed.) *The Body in Nursing*, Churchill Livingstone, Melbourne

Parker, J.M. and Gardner, G. 1991–92, 'Making ordinary: The nurse's voice', *Border Crossing, Meridian*, La Trobe University English Review, vol. 10, no. 2, pp. 71–8

——1992, 'The silence and the silencing of the nurse's voice: A reading of patient progress notes', *The Australian Journal of Advanced Nursing*, vol. 9, no. 2, pp. 3–9

Parker J.M., Gardner, G. and Wiltshire, J. 1992, 'Handover: The collective narrative of nursing practice', *The Australian Journal of Advanced Nursing*, vol. 9, no. 3, pp. 31–7

Parry, A. 1991, 'A universe of stories', *Family Process*, March, vol. 30, pp. 37–54

Probyn, E. 1993, *Sexing The Self: Gendered Positions in Cultural Studies*, Routledge, London

Prouse, M. 1995, 'A study of the use of tape-recorded handovers', *Nursing Times*, vol. 1991, no. 49, pp. 40–1

Revill, G. 1993, 'Reading Rosehill community, identity and inner-city derby', in M. Keith and S. Pile (eds), *Place and the Politics of Identity*, Routledge, London

Sacks, O. 1984, *A Leg to Stand On*, Pan Books, London

—— 1985, *The Man who Mistook his Wife for a Hat*, Pan Books, London

—— 1990, *Awakenings*, Pan Books, London

Sandelowski, M. 1991, 'Telling stories: Narrative approaches in qualitative research', *Image: Journal of Nursing Scholarship*, vol. 23, no. 3. pp. 161–6

Sawicki, J. 1991, *Disciplining Foucault: Feminism, Power and the Body*, Routledge, New York

Scheper-Hughes, N. and Lock, M. 1987, 'The mindful body: A prolegomenon to future work in medical anthropology', *Medical Anthropology Quarterly*, vol. 1, no. 1, pp. 6–39

Seymour, W. 1989, *Bodily alterations, An introduction to a sociology of the body for health workers*, Allen & Unwin, Australia

Silverman, K. 1984, 'Psychiatric discourse and the feminine voice', in C.S. Vance (ed.), *Pleasure and Danger*, Routledge and Kegan Paul, Boston

Smith S. and Watson J. (eds) 1992, *De/Colonizing the Subject, The Politics of Gender in Women's Autobiography*, University of Minnesota Press, Minneapolis

Sontag, S. 1990, *Illness as Metaphor and AIDS and Its Metaphors*, Doubleday, New York

Spreen Parker, R. 1990, 'Nurses stories: The search for a relational ethic of care', *Advances in Nursing Science*, vol. 13, no. 1, pp. 31–40

Street, A. 1992a, *Cultural Practices In Nursing*, Deakin University Press, Geelong

—— 1992b, *Inside Nursing: A Critical Ethnography of Nursing*, State University of New York Press, New York

Taylor, B. 1994, *Being Human: Ordinariness in Nursing*, Churchill Livingstone, Melbourne

Thurgood, G. 1995, 'Verbal handover reports; what skills are needed?', *British Journal of Nursing*, vol. 4, no. 12, pp. 720–2

Turner, B.S. 1984, *The Body and Society: Explorations in Social Theory*, Basil Blackwell, Oxford

—— 1992, *Regulating Bodies: Essays in Medical Sociology*, Routledge, London

REFERENCES

Van Manen, 1990, *Researching Lived Experience: Human Science for an Action Sensitive Pedagogy*, State University of New York Press, New York

Walker, K. 1993, 'On what it might mean to be a nurse: A discursive ethnography', unpub. doctoral dissertation, La Trobe University, Melbourne

——1994a, 'Confronting "reality": Nursing, science and the micro-politics of representation', *Nursing Inquiry*, vol. 1, pp. 46–56

——1994b, 'Research with/in nursing: "Troubling" the field', *Contemporary Nurse*, vol. 3, no. 4, pp. 163–8

——1994c, 'Toward a critical ontology: Nursing and the problem of the modern subject', paper delivered at the National Conference, *Foucault: The Legacy*, July 4–6, Ramada Hotel, Surfers Paradise, Queensland

——1995, 'Nursing, narrativity and research: Toward a poetics and politics of orality', *Contemporary Nurse*, vol. 4, no. 4, pp. 156–63

Webb, C. 1992, 'The use of the first person in academic writing: Objectivity, language and gatekeeping', *Journal of Advanced Nursing*, no. 17, pp. 747–52

Webster Barbre, J. et al. (personal narratives group) (eds) 1989, *Interpreting Women's Lives: Feminist Theory and Personal Narratives*, Indiana University Press, Bloomington

Weedon, C. 1987, *Feminist Practice and Poststructuralist Theory*, Basil Blackwell, Oxford

Wendall, S. 1996, *The Rejected Body, Feminist philosophical reflections on disability*, Routledge, USA

White, J. 1991, 'Feminism, eating and mental health', *Advances in Nursing Science*, vol. 13, no. 3, pp. 68–80

White, M. 1992a, 'Family therapy training and supervision in a world of experience and narrative', in D. Epston and M. White, *Experience Contradiction, Narrative and Imagination: Selected papers of David Epston and Michael White 1989–1991*, Dulwich Centre Publications, South Australia

——1992b, 'Deconstruction and therapy', in D. Epston and M. White, *Experience Contradiction, Narrative and Imagination: Selected papers of David Epston and Michael White 1989–1991*, Dulwich Centre Publications, South Australia

Whitford, M. 1991, *Luce Irigaray: Philosophy in the Feminine*, Routledge, London

Wilcox, H., McWatters, K., Thompson, A. and Williams L. (eds), 1990, *The Body and the Text; Helene Cixous, Reading And Teaching*, St. Martins Press, New York

Wiltshire, J. and Parker, J. 1996, 'Containing abjection in nursing: The end of shift handover as a site of containment', *Nursing Inquiry*, vol. 3, pp. 23–9

Wolf, N. 1990, *The Beauty Myth*, Vintage, London

Wolf, Z. 1986, 'Nurses' work: The sacred and the profane', *Holistic Nursing Practice*, vol. 1, no. 1, pp. 29–35

INDEX

abnormality, 97
alien body, 66
alternative therapeutic approaches, 119
ANCI competencies, see Australian Nursing Council Inc. competencies
anorexia, 67, 69, 71, 98
anti-depressants, 102, 104
anti-narrative, 33
artificial feeding, 71–2, 123–4
asthma, vi, vii, 2, 3, 40, 47, 83, 86–7, 114, 123
asthmatic, 85, 95, 110
Australian Nursing Council Inc. competencies, 10

basic nursing care, 49, 50–6, 83
binary logic, 26
busy nurse, 29

Capra, F., 8, 104

Cartesian, 7–9, 14, 16, 18, 22–3, 27, 36–8, 45, 75, 79, 85, 96, 99–100, 117, 134–5
Cataract Gorge, 3, 4
Christmas, 70
chronic fatigue syndrome, 100, 117
chronic illness, 119, 131, 133
chronicity, 111
confidentiality, 29, 50–1
crisis of representation, 31, 33

death, 71, 124–7, 132–3
depression, 102–3, 125
Descartes, R., 8, 16–17
diet, 62–3, 69, 71–2
dieting, 62–3
dietitian, 67–8
disease talk, 19
disembodied, 21, 53, 61, 68, 73, 75, 87
docile bodies, 40, 42, 46, 77

Index

Duck Reach, 4, 137
dying, 125, 128, 132–3

eating, 63–7
embarrassment, 91
embodiment, 6–7, 11, 33, 53, 69, 72–3, 79–82, 87, 89
enculturation, 52–3
euthanasia, 127, 133
exercise and diet, 2–3, 62
experts, 45

fear of fat, 2–3
first person, 33
Fonda, J., 69
food, 62–9, 71–2
Foucauldian, 53
Foucault, M., 14, 29–30, 42–7, 58, 61, 63, 96–9
fragmentation of care, 115–16
Frank, A., 17–22, 60, 101, 103, 128
Freud, S., 96

good patient, 48

handover, 10, 43, 50–1,
holism, 16
holistic, *see* holism
Holmes, C., 15
hopelessness, 116
Horsfall, J., 98, 102–3
hysterical conversion reactions, 96, 99

ICU, *see* Intensive Care Unit
Intensive Care Unit, 5, 40–6, 66, 87, 134

kingdom of the sick, 1, 38, 134

Klienman, A., 17–18, 103

Lawler, J., 6, 15–17, 50, 52–3, 79, 88, 91
Lumby, J., 10–11
Lupton, D., 62, 64–6, 68, 70

marginality of nurses, 29
Martin, E., 92
McInerney, F., 64
McLaren, P., 13–14, 23, 30
meaning making, 27
mechanical body, 7, 10, 47, 135
mechanics of power, 42, 45
medical,
  box, 109
  gaze, 43–5, 58
  narrative, 28
  restitution narrative, 125, 127
  salvation, 108
medicine, discourse of, 52, 58, 61, 135
menstruation, 91–2
mental health, 97
metaphysical, 90
mind/body, 25, 74–5, 78–9, 84, 95, 101, 104
Moore, T., 17–22, 60, 118
muscle weakness, 83–4
myalgic encephalomyelitis, 117

narrative, 6, 11–13, 19–21, 24, 28, 30, 33–4, 50, 86, 124–5, 135
  remembering, 28
  wreckage, 21
neuropsychological
  disturbances, 96
nursing, discourse of, 30, 52

nursing home, 120
nutrition, 40, 62, 64, 66, 68–9, 72, 126

object body, 7
objectification, 19, 45–6, 57, 78–9, 83, 111, 134
objectivity, see objectification
ontological crisis, 84
oppression, 52
oral culture, 10–11, 29
organic paralysis, 96

pain, 32, 82–3, 125
panoptican space, 43
Parker, J., 9–10, 50–1, 53, 79
passive patient, 46
phenomenology, 29
postmodern, 12, 20, 25
power/knowledge, 47
primary nurse, 60, 105–6
psych consult, 95, 98, 104
psychiatric patient, 105, 108–9
psychiatrist, 97, 103–4, 109, 125–6
psychiatry, 95–6, 98–9, 102–5, 109
psychogenic, 93
psychology, 96–7, 99, 102
psychosomatic, 9, 23, 76, 94, 96, 99–101, 107, 111, 114, 131
psychotherapy, 99

reductionism, 11
reductionist, 135
re-embodied, 75
regimes of truth, 30

rehabilitation, 107, 113–17, 119–20, 129
  definition of, 116
rejected body, 98
reliability, 32
restitution narratives, 125, 128
re-storying, 27, 30
rigour, 32

Sacks, O., 6, 17–22, 34, 60, 85–6, 89, 90, 96, 105, 136
science, discourse of, 79, 135
situating self, 19–20, 25, 33–4
social voice, 67
somology, 6
Sontag, S., 19, 23, 107, 124, 127, 133, 137
spinal injury, 120
storytelling, 6, 10–11, 19–20, 25–32, 36, 125
Street, A., 29, 52–4, 60
subjectivity, 23, 26, 32, 63, 72
surveillance, 43–4, 54

Turner, B., 14
therapeutic, 34, 55
third person, 32
totalising stories, 27
truth, 32, 44

validity, 18, 26, 32

Walker, K., 10, 29–34, 43, 111
wellness, 1
Wendall, S., 100–1, 117, 119, 121
wounded storyteller, 19, 21